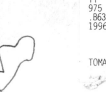

Plaited Glory

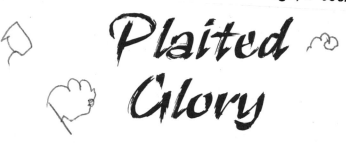

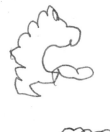

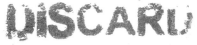

Also by Lonnice Brittenum Bonner

Good Hair

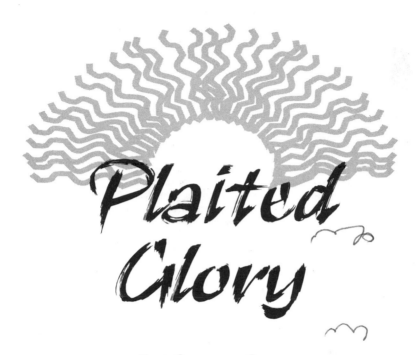

Plaited Glory

For Colored Girls Who've Considered Braids, Locks, and Twists

Lonnice Brittenum Bonner

THREE RIVERS PRESS • NEW YORK

For Derek and Roland

Published by Three Rivers Press, New York, New York.
Member of the Crown Publishing Group.

Random House, Inc. New York, Toronto, London, Sydney, Auckland
www.randomhouse.com

THREE RIVERS PRESS is a registered trademark and the Three Rivers Press colophon is a trademark of Random House, Inc.

Printed in the United States of America

Design by Mercedes Everett

Library of Congress Cataloging-in-Publication Data
Bonner, Lonnice Brittenum.
    Plaited glory : for colored girls who've considered braids, locks, and twists / by Lonnice Brittenum Bonner.
    Includes bibliographical references.
1. Braids (Hairdressing). 2. Hairdressing of Afro-Americans. I. Title.
TT975.B63   1996   646.7'245'0899673—dc20   96-4108

ISBN 0-517-88498-4

10 9 8

Contents

Acknowledgments

Jameela Al-Nafis

Raziya Al-Nafis

Diane Bailey, Tendrils Braiding Salon, Brooklyn, N.Y.

Aurelio Jose Barrera

Manie Barron

Olive Lee Benson, Olive's Salon, Boston, Mass.

Martha R. Blanding

Mary R. Blanding

Mrs. Nellie M. Bonner

Capril Bonner-Thomas

Maya Bonner-Thomas

Hajar Bonner-Thomas

Lawrence Braxton

Lonnie and Dorothy Brittenum

Laura J. Brooks

Thea Cook

Beatrice Dozier-Taylor

Tammerlin Drummond

Cecilia Hinds, Uzuri Braids, Washington, D.C.

Constance Melton, International Braiders Network, Brooklyn, N.Y.

P. J.

Chauser Perkins Trass

Special thanks and appreciation to Barbara Lowenstein, Norman Kurz, and all the associates.

And thank you, Carol Taylor, for your faith in my vision.

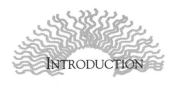

Signifyin' Hair

Start talking about braids, twists, or locks and the conversation can go almost anywhere. Countrified trail braids or gangsta plaits. Dreadlocks or cultivated salon locks. Braid weave perpetrating a straightened hairstyle. Ghetto or bourgie. Long supple braids or another fried do. Hair like silk or a bunch of nappy plaits. Hair that is saying something. Signifying hair.

It has been said that hair can communicate a great number of things and that people tend to make judgments based on appearances. No one seems to take that more seriously than African-Americans. Sometimes, in fact, it is taken too seriously, so that matters of choice, enjoyment, or simple practicality are no longer a consideration.

Women should be able to wear their hair in any manner that they choose—straightened, curled, crimped, waved—and if you have coiled African hair, the options should include Afrocentric styles. It is possible to manipulate your appearance in a manner that enhances your hair's natural attributes yet allows you to be presentable in this society. After all, America is about taking the best of what various cultures have to offer and making them part of the mix.

Braids evoke a mixed bag of feelings in African-Americans. Some people think that braids and all their variations are so ugly that they wonder why anyone would want to "go back to that." For them it is not an issue of expressing one's individual style or even respecting another's right to choice. Rather, there is only a special shame associated with having a racial feature that was held up to ridicule because it refused to disappear into the melting pot. "Can't we just move beyond that?" Well, I've tried, but my coils always seem to catch up with me, so I've learned to enjoy them. When I want a change, I take out my blow-dryer and change it. It's not a big deal anymore. Braids, twists, locks, and all their interpretations are part of our contribution to American style and culture. That's just the way it is.

I find it interesting to see how African-American styles have been translated from their African origins. Wrapping and threading are ancient hairdressing methods that originated in Africa, before history was recorded. When Africans were first brought to these shores, wrapping and braiding were among the arts that they continued to practice. Enslaved Africans took string from discarded clothing and used it to thread the hair. Sometimes rags were the best they could get.

My son's grandmothers, daughters of the South, remember seeing women wrap children's hair with yarn or colored strips of rags. The hair was sectioned into decorative and sometimes intricate partings. Each section was wrapped in yarn from the root to the end, until it resembled a long colored stick. The "sticks" would then be fashioned into styles like little yarn-covered knobs or loops. The hair of older girls was often wrapped with black thread. Women used threading to straighten the hair. Today, you can buy thread used to attach hair weaves and use it for threading.

Our mothers remember that when they were growing up young girls wore their hair underbraided and overbraided. Today, the underbraiding technique is commonly used to create Goddess Braids, and overbraiding can be seen in cornrowed styles. But forty or fifty years ago, both under- and overbraiding were quite popular methods for cornrowed styles for children. Black women who had a lot of hair or braided hairpieces could get away with Westernized versions of these styles—a crown or ring of large underbraids with bangs, for example—which were worn in the 1940s.

Many times a child's hair was parted into decorative designs and braided into a head full of small plaits. Each braid was tucked or braided into the subsequent one. These were called trail braids. Sometimes the plaits were left to hang free and a ribbon or barrette was used to adorn each plait. As a girl grew older (and mothers hoped that the hair grew along with everything else), the number of plaits was reduced, so that bigger girls had just two or three plaits, maybe four. This is an American interpretation of the way some African braided styles indicated the wearers' maturing status. To this day, mothers continue to adorn little heads in this manner.

The women of the Gabbra, a desert tribe in the Chelbi Desert of Kenya, wear cornrows parted down the middle and plaited into thick caps down to the neckline, with the ends left to curl up like a sort of braided flip. The women of the savanna tribes, like the Mali, Tuaregs, Fulani, and Bella, adorn their cornrows with beads, shells, coins, and even brightly colored buttons. The Senegalese people are noted masters of braiding, and the Southern Nigerians have highly developed threading techniques. Throughout Africa, braids range from the elaborate to the simple, which can mesh with Western fashions.

Many African hairdressing arts and techniques have been adopted by other cultures and much of the exchange occurred in colonized nations. French hairdressers in parts of colonized Africa, for example, adopted cornrow techniques and referred to them as "French braiding."

The more things change, the more things stay the same. "Silky dreads" or "silky locks" are African-American interpretations of African wrapping and threading techniques. It's interesting to note that with each wave of Afrocentric styles, the African vibe gets stronger and stronger.

I didn't grow up in a household that was particularly supportive of braids in any form. I suppose this was because my parents came from an era in which braids were either for small girls or were something to wear underneath a wig. Later on, as times progressed, my parents became more tolerant. But until tolerance arrived at our house, braids ranked below Afros. Remember, this was the time of The Revolution. Then there was Angela Davis. Sister Davis had the baddest Afro in the history of hairstyles. You must understand what a breakthrough that was. Before the Afro, the very idea that a black woman's African hair texture should be treated as an attractive, desirable asset was considered radical and offensive. So we sat up and took serious note of Sister Davis's 'fro. It was superbad.

But a lot of parents just couldn't dig it. First of all, how could this light-skinned child, with that *good* hair, just *waste* her looks like that? Second, we spent all this time coming up with the answer to The Problem—wigs and hair straighteners—and there she was, with a head full of naps. And third, all this talk about Black Power. Back in the day, people got their teeth knocked out for calling somebody black! Well, she could "go natural" if she wanted to, but *you'd* better not come in *this* house like that! And why were people bringing Africa into it? You weren't born in anybody's Africa!

After long deliberation, my mother finally consented to my wearing an Afro. But she insisted on calling it a "natural"—none of this Afro from Africa mess—and it had to be a "curly" one achieved by wrapping toilet paper around a million sponge curlers and rolling them up in my dampened hair. I'd fork it out with my pick—boy, I *loved* saying that. "Hey, girl, hand me my pick." It was like you belonged to this really cool race that had their own special combs. You'd be carrying your books to class. Your white girlfriend would have her brush on top of her stack— the better to smooth it through her bone-straight, Marcia Brady hair, which was all the rage—and your rake would be on top of your stack. For once, you felt good about having nappy hair. My first pick was the cheap small black one with the triangle handle with some black hair company's logo on it. Then I got Morrow's folding rake—the metal rake that folded into a plastic handle. Mine was black, of course. I never did get to the cake cutter stage, though; my 'fro wasn't mighty enough to really rate one. The cake cutter, a formidable, all-metal rake with a pearlescent plastic handle, was for the brother or sister with hair like the Sylvers. When it came time to rake it out, even the Jackson 5 had to step back and pay respect to the Sylvers. There were plenty of wanna-bes, though, with cake cutters stuck in Afros so thin that it seemed as if the rake was about to clatter to the floor, carrying the back of someone's kitchen with it.

It didn't take long to discover that a cake cutter was a formidable weapon and many schools began to outlaw them. Still, the censors overlooked a more subtle defense strategy. Before handguns in schools became commonplace, serious disputes were settled the old-fashioned way—by hand-to-hand combat. Cornrows were adopted as the ultimate in feminine battle chic. The idea was simple and effective: Cornrows made hair pulling more difficult.

Later on, a neighbor for whom I baby-sat gave me a dark brown Afro wig. The wig was cool with Mom because it was curly. Braids kinda went hand in hand with wigs because that was one way to get your nappy hair to lay down low enough to pin one on.

If you were lucky enough to have either a sister or mother who could really braid, you got cornrows. Nothing fancy, remember, this was going up under a wig. Parted in the middle, rows going straight down either side of the part. If your rows were done really neatly, you could get away with wearing it out and pinning on an Afro Puff in the back. Voilà! A hip new do! No, I didn't get any Afro Puffs, either. But I tried to simulate the look and was chastised by my mother for daring to expose the forbidden braids.

"Do I see you wearing those cornrows?" Mom asked, warming up for the close-in.

"Y-yes, ma'am." Just call me Gutless.

"Well, you can just take them out. I don't know why you want to wear plaits like that; they look just like little worms. Mama used to do my hair like that when I was little and I just hated them. I think they're ugly."

"Aww, Mommy, can't I wear them? Edna gets to wear *hers* to school."

"What did I say? And you'd better tuck those lips in."

I sucked my teeth and slunk off to my room. Revved up the old reel-to-reel and put on my *Cleopatra Jones* soundtrack. I chose the fight scene where Cleo puts her big 'fro up in an African headwrap and kicks Shelley Winters's booty (I recast my mom as Shelley) and took down my little cornrows.

I probably did look rough; my hair was on the thin side and I couldn't cornrow to save my life. The rows meandered down the sides of my skull in crooked lines and stopped well above my ears, which gave me that fashionable, balding look. My Puff was more like an Afro tennis ball stuck on the back of my head. But in my mind, I was ready for *Soul Train*.

I also used braids—plaits, actually—to blow out the old 'fro. Don't act like I'm the only one who was around when the Blowout was in circulation. Let's see, there was the standard method—braiding your hair up in little freestyle plaits or trail braids, where the end of each little plait was tucked into the beginning of the next one. Girls usually didn't want to be seen in public sporting what was considered to be a Farina look, so the braids replaced setting your hair at night. For boys, there was a whole new status angle to be exploited by getting a girl to braid up your hair on Saturday afternoon, so you could sport your biggest, fluffiest 'fro on Saturday night. Many brothers would wear their hair plaited up all week long, wearing wool watch caps to school, only to resurface with big hair on the weekend. The young gangsta factor took this to the extreme by wearing wool caps day in and day out, no matter how hot it was. The only time you saw hair was in the yearbook photo.

My parents believed that a young man should remove his hat when entering someone's home. It was a matter of respect and good manners. I couldn't figure out what disgusted them more, the thought of a roughneck with a lid on in their home or one with a head full of braids. It doesn't take much to imagine how this went down among the few brothers who ventured onto my doorstep. "It's Thursday, I just got my hair braided, and it's up under my hat. I'm here to check out Lonnice, a chick who I've heard hasn't given up any kind of play, nowheres, no how, and Pops is talking about me taking off my hat?" Homeboy and his hat spent about ten minutes on my doorstep before they moved on to a more permissive audience.

It took a while for corporate America to figure out that the natural was more than a brief fad and that people shampooed and groomed their hair while wearing them. The beauty industry kicked into gear with blowout combs, chemical kits, and Afro Sheen. The first combs were blow-dryer hybrids with picklike attachments. One particularly imaginative gadget was a hollow metal comb that blew out hot air and could allegedly double as a straightening comb, as the comb's head heated up to a temperature that could extend tight coils. The chemical blowout kits were mild-formula hair straighteners that promised to give you the curly, bouffant natural that everyone would desire. Special care had to be taken with the chemical blowouts or your Afro would turn into a wilted bush with a Moses part down the middle. Still, braids were by far the smarter method of cultivating the best natural.

I got another taste of braids while vacationing in Memphis. My cousin Natalie and her brother Nathan were both what I considered the Essence of Hip. I was in junior high and they were finishing college, but I hung on to every word they said. They were doing everything I longed to do—they drove cars, they shopped for clothes without their parents, they earned their own money, they stayed out late and didn't have to get permission for it. I was amazed to discover that the parties they went to didn't even *start* until ten o'clock. That was a totally new concept for me. Nathan wore a big 'fro that he'd blow out with braids. Natalie wore one, too, but one day she came home with a new do. I tuned in as she showed it off to the relatives, explaining that the name of the style came from its resemblance to little rows of corn. Cornrows! I was beside myself with glee. My mother had always thought well of Natalie and Nathan. They were both "sweet and well behaved." "I wouldn't mind if you turned out to be a little lady like Natalie," she'd say. I had it made in the shade, Jack. If Natalie was wearing braids, how bad could they be?

It turned out that cornrows were very bad for girls under twenty-one. One needed a certain maturity to wear them. Until then, one needed parental permission. When it came to justifying an argument, my mom could have put Thurgood Marshall to shame. But I didn't let that stop me from trying to coerce Natalie into braiding my hair anyway, in hopes that Mom would see the wondrous transformation of my Afrocentric beauty and be too moved to ask me to get rid of them. Natalie was like "No-o-o. Uh-uh. I don't want Aunt Dot upset with me." And so I had to admire them from afar. I would watch Natalie oil between the rows and smooth the plaits down before donning some large hoops done in silver wire to set off the look. How long . . . how lo-ong must I wait?

By the late seventies and early eighties styles had changed but my hair had not. Blow hair, that permed hair with the silky, "blow-in-the-wind" quality, ruled and I worked hard to get it. Sometimes my hair cooperated but it was a constant struggle. I was attending a university in Los Angeles by then and I began to see braids come back in. It was the era of the extension. Braid shops crept up all over L.A. You could get cornbraids, individuals all with that long, flowing look of long flowing hair. The cornrows were sold in layers. Layers were for the woman who couldn't afford individuals but wanted the look of a lot of hair.

Times weren't the only thing that had changed about me. Despite my admiration for cornrows in my youthful innocence, maturity and worldliness had begun to close in. It was the fear of Afrocentricity. Would I be able to get a boyfriend with my hair *like that?* What would people think? Could I get a job with my hair *like that?* Would I be allowed to graduate? Would the sky fall in? I asked friends what they thought about braids. Should I or shouldn't I?

One day, when I was supposed to be studying, I saw a trailer for a movie, a Blake Edwards film titled *10*. The clip featured a young white woman doing a slo-mo jog on the beach. She had blond hair done up in long braids. Not Heidi milkmaid braids. Beaded, soul sister braids.

Here I was, whining and deliberating about what people would say if I got my hair braided and some homegirl had literally run off with the prize. Many black women resented the success of Bo Derek's braids because it seemed that Afrocentric styles had to be validated by whites before they were considered fashionable. Others simply viewed it as sincere flattery. I viewed it as the proverbial "slap upside the head," a wake-up call. I got my braids and they were everything I'd imagined they would be.

I was watching *Sesame Street* with my son one morning and had the pleasant surprise of seeing a sketch called "The Braid-y Bunch." It was a takeoff on the opening credits and theme song of that popular seventies sitcom *The Brady Bunch*. In this case, Carol and Mike were played by a little African-American girl with cornbraids and a Caucasian girl with two long plaits. The black girl introduced her three friends, who had individuals, braids, and cornrows. The white girl brought on her girls, whose hair was done in French braids and plaits. I could only think about how I would have felt if something this cool had been on when I was a little tyke in dookie braids. Something that helps young people relate to their similarity, yet appreciate the diversity in their beauty. Now, *that's* what I call "moving beyond all that."

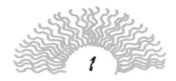

Parental Guidance Advised

What do you do with your child's hair? To perm or not to perm is the big question. Mothers who sport unprocessed locks are often the ones who are most frustrated when their daughters pester them for the latest fried-out do. There are many people who swear that chemical straightening is the easiest way to manage the unmanageable, but I have got to stand up for the children on this one. It's only easier if you are willing to put the same energy into your child's hair that you put into your own. And even then it still ain't easy. If you're a lady who is losing the battle for your own hair, chances are good that your daughter's hair will become another casualty.

You say you've had it with the early-morning hair wars, struggling through all those thick unruly coils that are making you late for work. "I'm gonna get that child a perm!" Problem solved.

Nothing can solve those pesky hair problems like a good chemical straightening. That was the dilemma of Sheila D. and her ten-year-old daughter, Iris, whose names have been changed at their request. The child had hair that most little and big girls would die for: enough to put into one long plait, a braid as thick as her wrist and fulla coils.

"I just run a warm comb through every week, and in the summer when she swims I have it braided," said Sheila, beaming. I remember thinking that this Iris is a sho' nuff poster child, and if her mother kept up the program, she could possibly finish high school with a full head of hair.

The last time I saw little Iris, her hair looked a lot straighter. It looked a bit thinner. Sheila was still working the long single braid, the front crowned with two barrettes, but there were now inch-long broken hairs standing up well past the hairline. A hairline that had a telltale reddish tinge and some nappy roots. Relaxer Revenge was beginning to creep in. What happened to the warm comb, the braids, her pride?

"I just got tired of dealing," said Sheila. "I started taking her to Ebay and he blah, blah, blah . . ." Her voice just kinda faded into noise because as far as I was concerned, Iris's hairline was saying all that needed to be said.

When Sheila finally got down to brass tacks, my hearing began to come back. It seems that when girl children have been blessed with an abundant head of hair, folks are eager to offer solutions to a troublesome problem, which they disguise as counsel. Sheila's counselors were her mother, Mrs. C., followed by style-master Ebay. Sheila casually mentioned that Iris's hair was looking a bit knotty and was about to freshen it up when Moms seized the opportunity. It seems that Momma C. was relieved to hear Sheila actually confirm what everybody knew all along—that Iris's hair was indeed nappy—but she hadn't wanted to dignify gossip by embarrassing her baby with direct questions. But here was Easter coming up and there was her little grandbaby looking like an orphan who lost her comb. Now that it was out in the open, there was no time to waste. Get Iris over to Ebay at Pony Express. If he couldn't do it, there were plenty who would.

Sheila resisted for a while. Then she thought she'd let Ebay give her a break and plait Iris's hair. The most she'd let him do would be to run a warm comb through it. He'd been taking care of Sheila for years now, and whenever her hairline began to creep away, Ebay could always stage a comeback. Ebay would take care of it. Ebay's solution?

"Run a warm comb—through *this*? This calls for a haaard press! You know I've got my hands full in this shop and I don't have time to be sweatin' over nobody's hair. What do you think a Kiddie Kit is for?"

I think it takes a certain strength of character to resist the popular mythology that a young child's hair not only looks better but is more easily managed when chemically straightened. Children themselves are bombarded with peer pressure from unenlightened friends and classmates who are ashamed of Afrocentric styles, primarily short Afros, African locks, or anything that reveals unprocessed hair that is tightly coiled.

Hair-care companies are aggressively marketing chemical straighteners for children. Be aware that it's still calcium hydroxide (the so-called "no lye") and sodium hydroxide (lye) that's doing the straightening, the same ingredients that are in the grown-up stuff. Kiddie lye preparations are still lye, so take care.

Many parents figure perms are easier to manage, but a child must be taught how to take care of chemically straightened hair and this is not as easy as it sounds. Maintenance means trims, conditioning, tying it up at night with silk scarves. Playground antics, sandboxes, rainy days with no umbrella, or the occasional food fight is sure to test the hardiest kiddie perm.

There's no sense in straightening a child's hair only to let it go because you can't make time for regular hairdressing appointments. I was reminded of this recently upon seeing two little girls accompany their father to the CVS drugstore in crisp white blouses, private-school plaids, and two of the most played-out perms I'd seen in a long time. Their little greased pony spikes—no tails here, just spikes—were edged by a dry ring of unprocessed hair. This ring extended at least an inch into the hairline, so both girls looked as if they had Bozo crowns. (No disrespect meant to Bozo; his hair never looked this bad.) Why folks continue to believe that badly done straight is better than the most well-groomed short natural is beyond me. Their father looked as if he had the means to send his daughters to a good school, and with the exception of their hair, the girls looked well cared for. I could only think of how the girls must have felt; I'll bet each of them would have readily traded the sharp uniforms for a pretty head of hair.

Young girls want to be stylish, and after a certain age, say the preteen years, you'll have to relinquish some restrictions. My suggestion is to instill a foundation in Afrocentric styling or managing the hair without radical chemical processing first, so the child will have a rudimentary knowledge of how to deal with her hair in the natural state. Like learning the alphabet first before learning to read. Then when the young lady becomes of age and wants to get the latest, she'll at least know how to care for her hair properly. When she has matured a bit, she will be able to make style decisions that won't cost her a head of hair, and even if she wants to wear chemically straightened styles, she won't lose her hair over them. You can't win all battles, and keep in mind that at some point, your daughter will have to make her own groom-

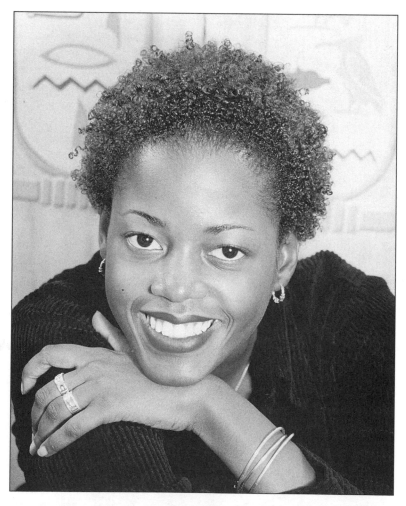

Jameela has that special allure that comes from a new attitude and a chic, natural do. Puts a whole new spin on those short hair hang-ups.

ing decisions. Just equip her with the education she needs and she'll make the right choices for her.

It was interesting to see this line of thinking in action when I met a mother who has worn her hair Afrocentrically for more than fifteen years. Raziya is a locktician on the West Coast and her daughter, Jameela, is an aspiring model in her early twenties.

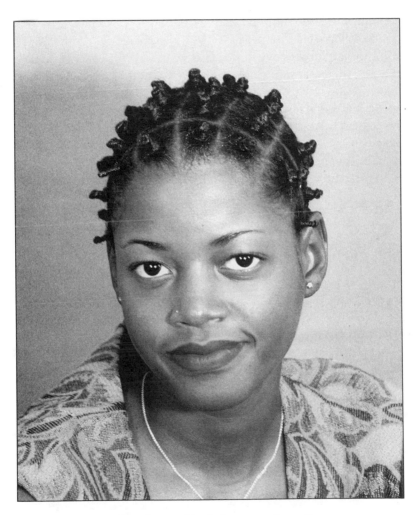

Nubian knots add a little spice to her coils.

Raziya said she herself had been through just about every straight do and curly perm in existence before settling into the real deal. Her locks are gorgeous. So when she told me she had a daughter, I couldn't wait to ask her how she wore her hair. She showed me some pictures. The prom picture: There was Jameela in a permed Hollywood do, dressed to kill. Jameela, in another snapshot, reclining on the floor, hair in the same perm—pretty girl, but looking kinda commonplace. Then she showed me recent pictures of Jameela. The perm was gone, and cropped coils framed glowing skin and a sexy smile. This wasn't even the same person. Those other snapshots looked like wish-me, wanna-be. The new Jameela looked like a contender. I wanted to know what had made Jameela come out of the perm. Raziya said that her daughter had realized that she needed that extra allure that Afrocentric hair could give her.

"Her true beauty emerged," Raziya said.

Eight-year-old Maya is blessed with a head full of extremely

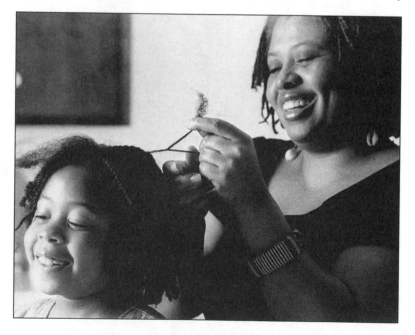

Maya is happy about getting her hair twisted because it doesn't hurt and it looks cute. Capril's happy because it lasts for three weeks.

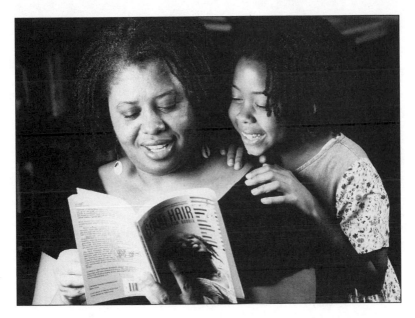

Maya's twists are done, Capril's locks are fierce. That leaves plenty of time for mother-daughter activities.

thick, healthy hair. Her mother, Capril, described Maya's hair as being so springy that it can stretch well past her shoulders, but retracts down to about three inches when wet. That's what is called supercoily hair. The kind of hair that ladies bitterly complain about and then wish would come back after they've burnt it off trying to make it "manageable." Capril has resisted chemically straightening both her daughters' hair. Maya prefers twists and her twelve-year-old sister, Hajar, prefers braids and cornrows at the moment.

Maya's individual twists take about ninety minutes to do and they can last up to three weeks without shampooing. Capril uses different oils and lubricants for twisting; Aveda's Humectant Pomade is her current favorite. Maya usually reads a book or watches a video while Moms tends to her coiffure.

Miss Maya is a stylish little sista with a mature outlook when it comes to her hair. She enjoys being unique. I asked Maya if she had ever had her hair straightened.

"Yes, Sugar [her grandmother] did our hair for Easter, but

it was too hot and it touched my ear," Maya said. "That hurt."

Would Maya get her hair pressed again?

"No, because I like my hair the way it is," she said. "I might get some locks later, but I like it this way right now."

With the burning question (couldn't resist that one) now settled, Maya revealed that her favorite style is individual twists. She either wears them falling naturally around her face or pulled up into a ponytail with the back loose. She is also fond of hats— a gold-and-brown crocheted African cap and two that Sugar made for her, one with a chic black brim and the other a black-and-white cap with a pompon on top.

Maya said she hasn't had too much flak about her hair from her classmates and friends. They like her hair because it looks good and it doesn't need extensions. But one time her roots were a little puffy and it was time for a retwist. One of her girls felt compelled to speak out.

"She said my hair looked like a spider," Maya giggled.

I asked Maya what she does when it rains.

She wears a jacket with a hood, she said, so matter-of-factly that I became unnerved. I flashed back to my own childhood. Most of my grammar school career was spent toting a folded-up raincoat to school—my mother had declared war on moisture in any form and my hair wasn't "going back" without a fight. So, to my ears, this "jacket with a hood" business sounded too good to be real.

"Wait a minute," I said. "Don't you wear one of your hats or carry an umbrella?" Grab a plastic bag, make a hat out of some notebook paper, batten down your hatches, sound the alarm . . .

Maya just gave me a look.

"It's only hair," she said.

Most parents quickly learn that children usually choose the opposite of what they themselves prefer, if only to show independence. If you are firm but matter-of-fact about it, children can't help but absorb your positive feelings about the hair they were blessed with, and it is bound to have some effect on them later on. Perhaps your daughter will surprise you with interest in Afrocentric styles, especially if she sees other girls her age wear-

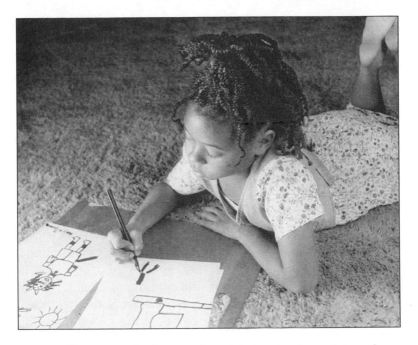

Maya likes to wear her hair up when she's deep into her artistic mode.

ing unstraightened styles that are appealing. On the other hand, don't be disappointed if she chooses a chemically straightened or processed style. (If she does, though, you still may want to encourage her to use Afrocentric styles such as braiding to give her hair periodic respites from chemically dependent styles.)

Baby Hair

If you're still wondering why kids develop hang-ups about the texture of their hair, check out parents and babies. Some women go as far as avoiding certain foods during their pregnancies— chitterlings and pork chops, to name a couple—just so their babies might have a certain texture of hair. As soon as a child is born, parents examine the hair and skin color. If an infant is born with a head full of soft, loosely curled hair, folks become very excited. They comb and brush it to death or put little ornaments on it or just sit around talking about how pretty it is. Then the predictions begin: Will he keep this wondrous gift or will it—gulp—will it *turn?* Is there a way, any way at all, that he can keep the baby hair until he reaches adulthood? Some mothers refuse to cut the baby's hair for as long as possible—if they could hold out until the child leaves home, they would—in hopes that they'll keep that soft baby hair. I notice that babies with a head full of tight coils don't get this kind of attention. Children notice this, too.

Our son didn't have much hair when he was born, just some thin tufts on the top of his head and a generous dose of cradle cap. Though we thought he was the cutest baby in the world, we were on a hair watch from Day One. We didn't care what *kind* of hair he was going to have, we just wanted him to grow some. When it finally started, we were very excited ("It's coming in! It's coming in!")—until we noticed that nothing was coming in on the sides. The boy had grown a mohawk, except most of it was sitting in a tuft on the back of his head. We nicknamed him Mawgwa, after a warrior in *The Last of the Mohicans* who sported the same do. We'd photograph him in flattering lighting, but even Industrial Light and Magic couldn't disguise the fact that the boy had very little hair and a whole lot of cradle cap. So when we sent out pictures, we'd pass the cradle cap off as his hair. We'd write on the back, "It's really coming in thick now!"

It's hard for parents not to be anxious about their child's development. Dermatologists advise that the only care an infant's hair (if he has any) requires is that it be kept clean. Comb or brush it just enough to arrange it. If the scalp becomes dry, use a little almond or baby oil to keep it supple. Some folks use a little baby lotion. Then put the child in a cute hat and take it easy. When our baby grew into a toddler with a head of thick, tightly curled coils, we moved on to other parental concerns like potty training. I'd spray a little leave-in conditioner in his hair and chase him around the room trying to comb and pat his hair into shape. No big deal. When he became willing to sit still for a haircut, his grooming became much easier. It was a sensible solution to his hair care.

≋ Cradle Cap

This is the scaly, oily-looking dandruff that is seen on infant scalps. It's very tempting to try and brush it away or pick it out. Don't do it. I did it and it was a bad idea. The vigorous brushing will irritate the baby's delicate scalp and picking at it will create sores. Just keep the scalp clean with normal cleansing and gentle brushing or combing as you see fit. As the infant's scalp matures, the condition will go away. It's as simple as that. Folks may suggest oil treatments and other remedies and they may seem to be effective, but the flakes will probably come back. Try not to worry about it.

≋ "My Baby's/Little Girl's Hair Won't Grow . . ."

We've all witnessed this scene. The sides are short and the top is long or the front is short and the back is broken or worn off. Common causes of this are sleeping habits and natural growth patterns. Children's hair texture is immature until they are about seven or eight years old. They can grow and shed an average of two or three textures before that time. The hair is not shed all at once, obviously, but at various points in time, softer textures will be mixed with stronger, more mature hair. When the child sleeps on his or her sides or back, the softer hair will be rubbed away, and the area will appear shorter until the stronger textures come in. This is often a temporary condition seen in infants, toddlers, and very young children, but can be turned into a chronic problem when parents begin chemical straightening or hot-combing in a misguided attempt to "grow" the hair or make it look longer.

Too many of us are horrified at the thought of a little nappy-headed daughter with short hair. The popular rationale is "I don't want her to look like a boy." Many infants have an androgynous look, and even when the parent does everything but dye the baby pink or blue, folks still don't guess the correct gender. So the hair dilemma is rather pointless. If the baby has no sides or back, it's cute and funny. But when the baby becomes a little girl, the laughter stops.

When this is the case, parents usually cling to the hope that the rest of the little girl's hair will catch up with the "long" part (which is usually two or three inches at best), so the child ends up with jacked-up, wish-me hair. Sometimes parents don't even attempt to style the child's hair with any dignity; they just clamp the "long" part in a barrette and call it a day. This looks worse than the "ugly short hair" that the parents are so desperately trying to get away from. Some fathers, who don't participate in any other aspect of child rearing, will rise up and forbid mothers to trim what's left of the child's hair. Mothers say things like "Her hair just won't grow," as if that excuses them from caring for their daughters' hair in a competent manner. You know this is a shame.

Try This

If the shorter areas are long enough for braiding, by all means go for it. Take your daughter to a braider if you're not up to the job yourself. If she's a toddler who won't sit still, do her hair in stages.

If the sides are so short that she has a short Afro and the crown is "long," trim the crown so the difference in length is minimized. Same thing if the back of the head is Afro length and the rest of the hair is only two inches longer. The "long" hair is what's left of the previous texture and it, too, will be shed and replaced. Little girls look darling in cropped naturals with earrings and a pretty outfit. Buy cute little hats for her to wear. You can really work this, and your little girl can learn to have style, dignity, and self-respect. If you are worried that she'll be teased, look at it this way: Her hair looked wrecked before, so she was gonna get capped on, anyway. At least now her hair will be short and stylish. Once it's back on the growing track, she can get braids, twists, or whatever you both can agree on.

≈≈≈ Budgeting

Many mothers will spend a substantial amount of money in the salon, faithfully returning each week for a fresh do, but when it comes to the children, it's catch-as-catch-can or "Can you do fast and cheap?" Most parents understand that it's unwise to spend too much money on items that kids will quickly tire of or outgrow, and while the latest hairstyle may fall into one of those categories, children won't outgrow a foundation in proper hair grooming.

How many times have you seen this picture: a mama with a played-out perm and her child wearing thick, long, unstraightened plaits. The hair psychic predicts . . . a child whose hair is living on borrowed time.

How about this scene: blow-'n'-curled mama with a permed child wearing a head full of sponge rollers—in the daytime. This is a child with a woefully overprocessed head of hair, and Mama is trying to keep a curl in it. Then again, it could be the Saturday before Easter.

Children require upkeep. As a child, I swore I'd never utter the words "I'm not spending forty dollars on one pair of socks! I don't care if Ice Box is wearing them! You must think money grows on trees!" Then I became a parent. Figure out what you want to spend and make a reasonable budget. Here are some things to consider.

To Perm or Not to Perm?

When your daughter asks for those $300 Silky Locks, that $7 Kiddie Perm will look like a steal. Be honest with yourself; think of your child's hair. Are you prepared to do what's necessary to keep a perm in top shape? The conditioning, the touch-ups, the strand test? Do you really know how to use the perm or will you end up asking the hairdresser to give (weave) your baby some hair? What style is the child going to wear or are you just going to plait it up? Do you really need a perm just to plait it up?

Better Choice

Go Afrocentric for everyday wear, and use that warm comb when the child is begging for a change. Makes better sense dollar wise. Braids can be very practical for a young girl. Who says you have to get the $300 extensions? There are plenty of styles to choose from—two or three plaits, cornrows, twists, or whatever strikes your fancy.

A lot of styles will last about two weeks before they need shampooing. You could send your child to get her hair braided every two weeks just as easily as you'd send her to get it straightened, but with braids, you'd get to skip that morning hair workout and get other things done.

Budget Time for Hairdressing

You make time for *your* hair appointments, don't you? Be realistic about your children's hair needs, your skill, and your time. If you hate doing your own hair, please spare the hair of your child. Find a good braider—freelance or salon—for the child and patronize him or her.

If that doesn't work for you, nail down some simple styles that you can handle. Two fat cornrows with ribbons can be very presentable and last a couple of days at a time depending on the age of your daughter and how well she sleeps in a scarf.

See the illustrations for another style suggestion that you can do at home. It can last at least a week or maybe two.

Set aside a regular time for hairdressing. Wash and braid on Thursday nights, then you're free for the weekend and can give the hair a once-over for church. Figure out a schedule that works for you.

Make hairdressing a pleasant experience—"Be still so I can get this comb through your knotty mess! If your hair wasn't so bad, it wouldn't hurt so much!"

It only makes things worse if your children get the same derision and messages of self-hatred at home that they can find anywhere in the streets. Children are probably not going to stop teasing one another about having nappy hair, but think of how little the teasing would mean to a child who looked forward to having her hair braided because it looked pretty and her scalp massaged because it felt good. Give her pretty hair sticks and clips—she'll treasure them.

Help your child deal with peer pressure—If your children come home talking about "good" and "bad" hair, don't reinforce the notion. Instead, ask what they mean by good and bad hair and explain where the terms come from. Set them straight in a constructive but firm manner, and forbid them to use those terms in the future. Then let it alone, but let them see images in your home that reinforce the image of African hair and features—all shades and hair textures—as being desirable. The books and art in your home are a good place to start. Be persistent. Remember that your children aren't necessarily going to listen to what you say but they do watch what you do.

Use gentler methods of grooming—If your child's hair is tightly coiled, make combing a painless experience. Divide the hair into sections and moisturize before combing. You can use water or dilute some leave-in conditioner in a spray bottle. Sometimes commercial detangling sprays help, but not always. Read the next chapter, "Four Degrees of Preparation," for combing techniques and hair-grooming tips. Learn how to give your child a scalp massage. See the following page for an easy style suggestion.

Invest in your child's self-image—If you feed your daughter's self-esteem you'll raise a beautiful woman.

This style is a bun or puff ringed by individual braids or twists. You can adapt it to shorter hair by substituting wide cornrows for the individual plaits.

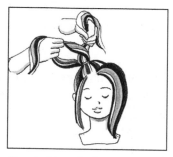

Fig. 1. *Part the hair over each ear in diagonals about three inches thick, as in the illustration. Pull back section up into a ponytail. You can braid it or make a bun or small Afro Puff.*

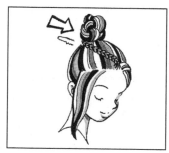

Fig. 2. *Part the hair in the smaller sections and braid into individuals or twists.*

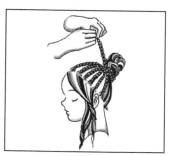

Fig. 3. *Anchor each braid or twist around the base of the large braid or bun.*

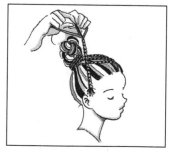

Fig. 4. *Do the same on the opposite section.*

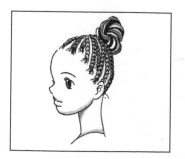

Fig. 5. *If you tie the braids up with a silk or satin scarf, this style should last for two weeks.*

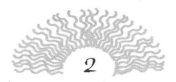

2

Four Degrees of Preparation

Before you put your hair into a sort of hypersleep, there are four things you need to do: shampoo and condition your hair, remove tangles, and lubricate the strands so they'll remain supple.

Think of braids and twists as being a spa for your hair, helping to preserve it for as long as possible during its growth cycle on your scalp. You've got to make sure it's well conditioned and supple. In this chapter I'll cover shampoos and conditioners, followed by how to prepare the hair for plaiting. Some salons and stylists will perform these services for you, but if you are seeing a freelance stylist, chances are that you'll be doing the prep yourself. Remember, if it's brittle when you put it up, it will break off soon after you take it down.

It used to be that whenever I read hair books and got to the part about "the parts of the hair are blah, blah, blah," I'd skip past it and get to the choice sections like the product recommendations and styles. Then, after I'd spent my meager cash on the products, I'd wonder why my hair continued to wither and break off. When I finally understood how hair is structured, though, I was able to jettison the hype and make product selections that were based on reality instead of desperation. You can do it, too.

African hair is not the headache you've been led to believe it is. It simply comes in varying degrees of curliness that range from loose waves to the tiniest coiled springs. The unique quality that sets our hair apart from that of other races is the degree of curliness.

Anatomy of a Hair

Check out the illustration of a hair strand. Each hair grows from a *follicle*, which is the pore from which the hair emerges. The root of the hair is called the *papilla*. When you pull out a hair, the whitish bulb you see is what remains of the papilla. Each hair follicle is nourished by a *sebaceous gland* that oozes an oily, waxy substance called *sebum*. If your hair feels dirty and you scratch your scalp, you can see the oily sebum underneath your fingernails.

The hair shaft itself is made up of three different layers of *keratin*, a fibrous protein. (Your fingernails and toenails are also made of keratin.) The outside layer is the *cuticle*. The cuticle is the hair strand's first line of defense against damage, like the shingles on the roof of a house. It contains the hair's pigment.

The layer underneath the cuticle is called the *cortex*. The cortex is a bunch of ropelike fibers that determine the thickness or thinness of your hair shaft. For example, women with fine, baby-soft hair have hairs with a thinner cortex, while women with coarse or wiry hair have thicker cortexes. Many women with thick hair mistakenly believe it is coarse because it is tightly coiled.

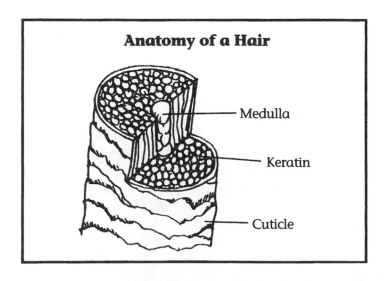

Anatomy of a Hair

— Medulla

— Keratin

— Cuticle

The middle or core of the hair shaft is called the *medulla*. It is a soft keratin layer.

〰 Curly, Wavy, or Straight

The shape of the individual hair shafts is what determines whether your hair is curly, wavy, or straight. Curly hair comes out of an almost flat-shaped follicle, straight hair comes out of a round follicle, and wavy stems from an oval follicle.

You can have curly hair with wavy sections or straight hair with some waves. There are many degrees of curliness in African hair, ranging from wavy to very tight, watchspring coils. If you pull out a strand of tightly coiled, unprocessed African hair, it will resemble a small coiled spring. Many women with African hair have two or three degrees of curl on different parts of their scalp. When I grew a head of unprocessed hair, I discovered that the curls on the crown of my head and nape of my neck were looser than those on the sides and back.

Where did this distinctive trait come from? There is evidence that the ancestors of people with lighter skins and straighter hair lived farthest from the equator, in cooler climates, and those with darker skins and curlier hair originated closer to the equator, with its intense heat and sun. Those who had more melanin in their

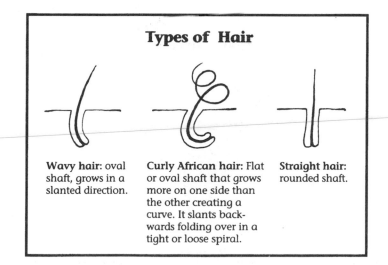

Types of Hair

Wavy hair: oval shaft, grows in a slanted direction.

Curly African hair: Flat or oval shaft that grows more on one side than the other creating a curve. It slants back-wards folding over in a tight or loose spiral.

Straight hair: rounded shaft.

skin survived longer because the skin was protected from chronic sun damage. The coiled hair stood away from the scalp and protected it from the sun while allowing air to flow through and cool the scalp. Then the African penchant for adornment took over and some groups chose to shave or crop their hair while others preferred a more elaborate presentation. It makes sense to me; I like the idea of form following function.

When I first read this, I thought to myself, Yeah, right. If our hair structure is so ingenious, why are so many black women struggling to keep it on their heads? Well, the truth is that when you alter structures, you have to compensate for the change because alteration affects function. Next I'll give you some familiar complaints, and when you take the hair's structure into consideration, it becomes easier to understand why things go wrong.

≈≈≈ "It's Dry"

Sebum, the oily, waxy substance originating in your hair follicles, works its way down the hair shaft to lubricate the hair. If your hair is *naturally* straight or loosely waved (emphasis on *natural* here), the sebum flows straight down, without any interruption.

Now visualize that oil coming down a shaft of coiled African hair. Instead of flowing down, it must work its way down every twist and turn of the coil. If the shaft is very tightly coiled, the oil doesn't make it to the ends without assistance—brushing and/or applying lubricants like oils or creams. Loosely curled hair has a better chance for oil distribution, but it still needs a little extra help. And so your hair feels dry, even when the scalp is oily. That's why oiling the scalp is less efficient than oiling the hair itself, particularly the ends. The exception to this is when the hair is braided; somehow the exposure of the scalp tends to make it a little dryer, so a plant- or vegetable-based oil used sparingly on dry areas does seem to help.

When my hair has been thermally or chemically straightened without adding oil, sebum would actually make it to the end of my hair strands. However, straightening is not a cure for dry hair. Chemical straightening breaks down the keratin bonds in the cuticle so the curls will straighten out. The loss of keratin and the chemical process make your hair shaft drier because the protective cuticle has been altered. Overprocessing, not an uncommon occurrence, destroys parts of the cuticle. You can also destroy your hair shaft if your pressing comb is too hot or you overdose on blow-dryers, hot curlers, and irons. At one time I was getting my relaxed hair pressed. Over a period of time, the ends of my hair split and turned white because the combination of blow-drying and pressing my relaxed hair was too much for my particular texture. My hair was bathed in sebum, but the solution was a trim and investigation of another styling method. So even though sebum can flow down straightened hair, it isn't enough to correct chemically or heat-induced damage.

≈≈≈ "It Doesn't Shine"

Light hits the shingles on straight hair and refracts off them the way light bounces off a pane of smooth glass. If your hair is tightly coiled, the light must reflect off the twists and turns, and the shiny effect is diminished. African hair can have a healthy gleam if it's in good condition, but the glow is more like that of fine suede than shiny patent leather. When you glop on the oil or heavy pomades in an attempt to get the same type of shine that women with naturally straight hair have, it looks greasy. It's better to apply a transparent color glaze or try one of the shine products containing silicone or dimethicone instead.

≈≈≈ "My Relaxed Hair Breaks and My Natural Hair Tangles"

When your hair is in bad condition or has been overprocessed, the cuticle shingles are roughened and broken. Sometimes parts of the shingle will be missing altogether. The opened cuticle of one strand catches onto the cuticle of another and the hair tangles. The inner layers of the hair strand are unprotected and it breaks easily.

Chemically processed hair is especially delicate when wet. When water hits the already weakened bonds, they become like limp strings. Wet, overprocessed hair has the consistency of overcooked pasta—limp and spongy.

Unprocessed coiled hair is better off in the tangle department than most women think. Left to their own devices, the curls coil around one another when your hair is dry. And each twist and turn is a weak spot in the hair shaft, so careless handling will encourage breakage. That's with *dry* hair. The bonus of unprocessed coiled hair is that moisture—that's water—softens it and makes it much easier to comb through or de-tangle.

In Search of . . . Shampoo

Whenever I hear someone insisting on the healing properties of a certain brand of shampoo or conditioner, I'm reminded of an old television show called *In Search of . . .* , which used to run on weekend afternoons, when most people had better things to do. The show's premise was a search for fabled people, objects, or places, like the Fountain of Youth. The narrator would drone over blurry footage of the alleged fountain. Then came the talking-head interviews with people who claimed they knew somebody who had actually visited the fountain and drank the water. If you lasted until the end, you'd be treated to highlights of next week's show, which promised, for example, a search for the Loch Ness Monster. Well, sign me up for the next expedition—I'll find the shampoo that will make hair weaves obsolete.

(I don't get into specific brand names in this book, other than to give examples of the type of product I'm referring to. I believe that you make better choices by knowing what your hair requires rather than by simply being given recommendations of brand names.)

≋ How to Choose a Shampoo

Shampoos are designed to clean your scalp and hair. Shampooing removes residues from oils and styling products from the scalp. It also opens the cuticle of the hair shaft, which prepares it for a conditioning treatment.

First, look for a shampoo that is pH balanced; most labels specify whether a shampoo is or not. The degree of alkalinity and acidity in the product is denoted by its pH. A pH of around 5 is close to that of your hair and scalp. If the shampoo is too alkaline, the cuticles of the hair will be more ruffled than usual and your hair will tangle easier.

Mild formulas are better for frequent shampooers because they won't strip away every bit of natural oil secreted by your scalp. Formulas with exotic vegetable and mineral additives do more for the promotion of the product than they do for your scalp, but indulging in them won't hurt you. I've tried baby shampoos in the past but found them to be very drying. I've since learned that this is because baby shampoos are designed to remove the heavy coating of sebum that coats the soft hair of infants.

Here are suggestions for shampoos based on hair needs, as well as descriptions of some other specialized shampoos.

Natural or Unprocessed Hair

Gentle shampoos that minimize dryness. Look for moisturizing formulas.

Chemically Processed Hair

Formulas designed for relaxed or waved hair are fine; moisturizing formulas are also good because chemically processed hair is usually on the dry side.

Color-Treated Hair

There are several brands that sell formulas for colored hair, or you can use any mild pH shampoo. The coloring process tends to leave the cuticle ruffled and this is what gives colored hair a more "full-bodied" look. It also makes the hair drier, so look for moisturizing qualities.

Buildup-Remover or Clarifying Shampoos

These shampoos will remove buildup of styling products, hard water, or other dulling, drying residues. These are good to use before coloring your hair because the color will "grab" better. They are also good if you've been doing a lot of swimming in chlorinated pools or the ocean. In fact, it's not a bad idea to use a buildup-remover shampoo once a month if you're in the habit of using a lot of products like gels, sprays, or pomades.

Balsam Shampoos

I avoid shampoos that contain balsam. Balsam is a resin that dries to a hard, clear film on the hair shaft. It feels good while you're washing and does soften the hair enough to de-tangle, but the balsam residue makes your hair drier later.

Shampoo-and-Conditioner Combos

The idea of a shampoo and conditioner combined sounds like a time-saver, but my hair always seems to benefit more from a *proper* conditioning treatment, like a shampoo that cleanses my scalp and hair, followed by a hot-oil treatment or a deep conditioner. I feel more secure with the traditional method. But if I were on vacation and had a choice between a combination shampoo/conditioner or no conditioner at all, or had no time for anything else, I'd go for it. If you use a shampoo/conditioning combo, it's a good idea to follow up with a leave-in conditioner. You'll read more about conditioners later.

≈≈≈ Flaky Possibilities

Everything that flakes is not dandruff. If you think you have dandruff, examine your scalp. Mild but annoying flaking could be the residue from styling products like gels or sprays. It can even be residue from conditioners that haven't been rinsed out properly. Petroleum- or mineral-based lubricants can also cause the scalp to flake because they tend to be irritating. For that reason, I've found that vegetable- and plant-based oils are best for hair and scalp care. Try clarifying shampoos or switching to other hair products than the ones you've been using before checking out dandruff shampoos.

Severe, heavy flaking and itching, accompanied by a reddened scalp and/or pus, requires a dermatologist's care.

There are several formulas on the market that have different effects, so please read the labels before you use them.

Keratolytic Shampoos

Contain sulfur or salicylic acid. This chemical dissolves the hair flakes. Let me remind you that sulfur stinks, so you will have an odor in your hair unless the label says otherwise.

Important! Avoid keratolytic shampoos if you have chemically processed hair. The sulfur reacts with the hair and causes it to mat, tangle, and break.

Cytostatic Shampoos

May contain tar, selenium sulfide, zinc pyrithione, or pyrithione zinc. These ingredients slow down the cell turnover that creates flakes. They can also be drying, and sometimes your scalp will overcompensate by producing too much oil. Some tar shampoos can discolor your hair if it's been lightened or bleached. Please read the labels.

Alpha Hydroxy Shampoos

Contain alpha hydroxy acids derived from fruit, sugar, or milk. AHAs exfoliate skin by sloughing off old, dull cells, thereby making the skin appear clearer. I have used an AHA hair/body cleanser and it does get rid of minor flaking, but I don't care for the way my hair feels afterward. So I use the AHA shampoo for the first lathering, rinse it out, then use a regular shampoo. I don't use AHA shampoos frequently, only when I notice a lot of flakes.

Conditioning

I used to be a product junkie. I whispered the latest brand name from the side of my mouth with the best of them. I could start a beauty-supply shop with all the shampoos and conditioners gathering mold in my shower caddy. I spent a lot of money to learn that the best conditioning treatment is preventive treatment.

≈≈≈ How Conditioners Work

Conditioners are designed to replenish the hair shaft with moisture and elasticity. They work best when the cuticle is open, as it is after a shampoo. Some conditioners help moisturize by replacing oils washed away by shampoos before smoothing the cuticle, creating a healthier appearance. After the conditioner has been absorbed, the extra residue is removed during the rinse and the cuticle should close. The cuticle can also be encouraged to close by rinsing the hair with water that has been acidified, as in an old-fashioned vinegar rinse. Cool water also encourages the cuticle to close.

Hair Beyond Repair

The only thing a conditioner can do for overprocessed or heat-damaged hair is to buy you a few minutes as you psychologically prepare yourself for the loss involved with getting a serious trim or haircut. There are products out there that claim they can do everything short of growing hair and I have used them. But if your hair is shot and you continue to abuse it, conditioners won't do anything for you but wear out your ATM card buying them.

Creme Rinses, Finishing Rinses, and Leave-In Conditioners

I've grouped the conditioners according to their purpose. As a general rule, chemically relaxed and/or colored hair needs moisture obtained from moisturizing conditioners or hot-oil treatments. Hair breakage caused by heat damage or chemical overprocessing requires an infusion of protein to temporarily bolster the cuticle. Most deep conditioners or protein formulas will do the job. In general, the rinses are used to de-tangle hair, by smoothing the cuticle and making it easier to comb. If you want to use them to control bushiness, you can double or triple the amount the manufacturer recommends. You don't need to spend a lot of money—the standard brands will do.

Leave-in conditioners are usually watery formulas designed to moisturize and/or prepare the hair for blow-drying or thermal styling. Many formulas feature herbs and oils. Some formulas close the hair shaft by acidifying the cuticle before coating it with a protective balm. If you must use the shampoo/conditioner combinations, a leave-in conditioner is a good way to finish your hair.

Instant Conditioners

These smooth the hair cuticle and de-tangle, with moisturizing or protein formulas that deposit a thin coating of hydrolized protein in the hair shaft. Instant conditioners usually remain in the hair from one to three minutes before rinsing. Manufacturers will offer different formulas for different hair types.

Deep Conditioners and Protein Conditioners

Deep conditioners give you a more intense conditioning treatment. The proteins are processed so they can penetrate the opened cuticle and enter the cortex to temporarily replace keratin loss caused by heat or chemical damage. Deep conditioning also helps seal in moisture. Most are left in the hair for about thirty to forty minutes, and it is recommended that during that time you apply heat, which helps open the cuticle even more and promotes the most intense absorption. There are several types of proteins that are commonly used to beef up conditioning treatments, usually derived from animal or vegetable materials.

Reconstructing Conditioners

The key words on these conditioners are "extremely damaged hair," but don't look for the miracles they promise because you and I both know it's only a matter of time before you'll be reaching for the trimming scissors. These contain complex proteins or nucleic acids that temporarily bond to the protein structure in your hair. Some heavy-duty professional formulas can be thick and syrupy, and a lot of the high-intensity protein formulas have a bit of a stink to them. Some formulas require heat but many don't. You should be extremely careful when using the formulas that dry into stiff helmets before they are rinsed out, *as you can lose hair if you don't remove all traces of the conditioner.*

Hair-Repair Conditioners

A lot of these formulas come in vials and have a thin, watery consistency. Some are used for a series of shampoos, after which the hair shaft is "repaired." But it's a temporary thang. They're betting that you probably won't understand.

≋ How to Choose the Right Conditioner for Your Needs

It's actually very simple.

Chemically processed hair is usually fighting breakage in addition to dryness, so you'll be dealing with the protein conditioners to rebuild what chemical processing removes and moisturizing to compensate for dryness. Hot-oil treatments are also good.

Natural or unprocessed hair needs moisture. You can get this through moisturizing conditioners or hot-oil treatments.

Thermal styling includes hot curlers, blow-drying, pressing, and bonnet dryers. Heat evaporates moisture, so compensate with moisturizing conditioners and hot-oil treatments.

≋ Conditioning Oils

Hot-oil treatments are the most efficient way of moisturizing and lubricating your hair. African hair thrives on oil. You can mix your own or buy commercial preparations if your pocket is flush. I like to splurge once in a while, but the idea of $15 for "eight [unspecified] natural oils" is hard to justify when I know exactly what kind of olive oil I can get from the supermarket for $3.50.

It's best to buy oils in quantities you know you'll use in a reasonable amount of time because oils will go rancid over time. You will also want to avoid using mineral- or petroleum-based oils on the scalp because they tend to clog pores and make the scalp flake and itch.

Rosemary oil is distilled from the herb rosemary. (If you cook pork, you know it's the herb you use to season a roast.) It's supposed to remove tangles and make your hair manageable. It's also inexpensive. It's been touted as a daily grooming aid, but when I uncapped it, the smell rushed out and knocked me back! It's extremely odoriferous; everyone will know you're using it until it quiets down. I like to mix it with a base of olive oil.

Olive oil, in my experience, is the most reasonable oil to use for conditioning. You can get it at just about any supermarket, and at three to four dollars for a twenty-five-ounce bottle, it's affordable. You can use it as a base oil combined with other oils like rosemary or vitamin E.

Sage oil has a clean, pungent smell like the herb from which it's distilled. The astringent quality soothes itchy scalp. It's inexpensive and can be purchased at health stores.

Jojoba oil is popular in hair-care products. It's supposed to be a good skin moisturizer and remove hardened sebum from the scalp. I haven't tried it on my face, but it works okay on my hair. For as much as it costs—I paid almost five dollars for two ounces—it didn't do as much as I thought it was going to do. One manufacturer even recommends using it as an aftershave. . . . What the heck, if you've got the bucks, most health-food stores have the jojoba.

Coconut oil is rather rich and fragrant. If you're on vacation in Mexico, the Caribbean, or most beach resorts, you'll discover local vendors often hawk coconut oil for a couple of dollars. Instead of frying your skin with it, buy some and use it as an inexpensive hot-oil hair treatment at the beach. Pure coconut oil tends to harden when it cools, so it may not be a good choice for everyday scalp care.

Castor oil is used in a lot of hairdressings marketed for men. It did an adequate job of lubricating the ends of my hair, but I found it to be kind of sticky and difficult to shampoo out. It also made my scalp flake.

Almond and sesame oils are also good choices to use for hair care.

All the oils mentioned can be found in health stores and some in supermarkets.

≋ How to Get Maximum Benefit from Conditioners

Condition your hair after shampooing while the cuticle is opened and the hair shaft can absorb an efficient amount.

Use a heating cap to help your hair absorb deep conditioners and hot-oil treatments. I bought mine at a beauty supply a few years ago. Heating caps are affordable and well worth the money.

Stock up on disposable plastic caps from the beauty supply and use them for conditioning treatments. You can also use plastic kitchen wrap in a pinch.

Learn to read labels. You don't have to be a chemist to under-stand what you are getting for your money. Ingredients are usu-ally listed according to their proportion in the formula. A typical first ingredient in many hair products is water. However, if you are choosing a reconstructive protein conditioner, you would want to see some sort of protein as the second ingredient. If pro-tein is way down on the list, I'd expect that product to be less effective than other brands. I'd also expect it to be a lot cheaper.

A cosmetic dictionary can turn out to be a good investment. I've used *A Consumer's Dictionary of Cosmetic Ingredients*, by Ruth Winter (Crown Publishers). Get the latest edition, and when in doubt, check it out.

Minimize or eliminate the use of heat to style your hair. If you don't have heat damage, you won't need to deep-condition so often. Use the lowest heat settings when blow-drying your hair. You can even dry your hair on a cool setting—it takes longer, but it saves your hair.

Concentrate on the ends of your hair because it's the oldest and driest part. If you're just about out of conditioner, be smart and use that last precious dab on the ends. The hair closest to your scalp is usually the healthiest, unless you've been blasting it with heat or chemicals.

Preparing to Braid

You've selected your shampoo, conditioner, and oils. If your hair is extremely damaged, you may want to plan out a conditioning regimen a few weeks before you're scheduled to braid. For exam-ple, you may want to do a deep protein conditioner a couple of weeks before you plan to braid and do a hot-oil session the week you have it braided. Your braider may have other suggestions along these lines.

≋ How to Shampoo Without Tangling Your Hair

I prefer to wash my hair in the shower because I can rinse more thoroughly. One of the best hair investments you can make is to buy a detachable showerhead. I use the Shower Massage, by Water Pik. A detachable showerhead allows you to rinse properly and thoroughly. It helps you wash your hair in a manner that minimizes tangling and matting. And it's affordable and easy to install.

If your hair is longer than four inches, use plastic clips to separate it into three or four sections before shampooing. Wet a section of hair and apply a quarter-sized dollop of shampoo. If your hair is very long, apply the shampoo to your scalp only and work down to your ends. Remember, the ends are drier and more porous and it doesn't take much to clean them or dry them out.

Work the shampoo through each section with the pads of your fingers. Move your fingers through your hair and scalp in one direction and you'll minimize tangling and matting. Washing your hair in sections makes it easier to get to your scalp and concentrate on loosening the dead scalp cells without hopelessly matting and tangling your hair in the process.

Rinse each section for at least one minute with very warm water and clip it out of the way. Finish with cool rinse water.

It may take up to three latherings for your hair to feel clean, but you don't have to clean until it squeaks. The exception to this is if you use a buildup remover or clarifying shampoo. These formulas tend to give you that squeaky-clean feel.

≋ The Squeaky Coil Gets the Oil

Hot-oil treatments are the best way to ensure that your hair will be supple. You can use the hot-oil treatment as a pre-shampoo conditioner or after shampooing. If your hair is to be plaited, I prefer the après-shampoo treatment.

Your hair should already be parted into three or four manageable sections after your shampoo. Towel-dry the sections so they remain wet but not dripping.

Warm up the oil of your choice. The amount depends on the amount of hair you have—one fourth to one half cup—but don't use so much that you'll need several shampoos to wash it out. Nuke it in the microwave for a minute or place it in a pan of hot water. Be sure and test the temperature on your wrist before putting it in your hair.

41

Apply the oil to your hair, section by section. You can use a cotton pad or your fingers. I prefer fingers because it seems like most of the oil is soaked into the cotton. Using my fingers allows me to smooth the oil down the hair strands and control it better. You can also massage a bit of the oil into your scalp while you're at it.

When you've evenly distributed the oil, loosely pile your hair on top of your head and cover it with a plastic cap or wrap. If you have the time, cover the cap with a towel and let your body heat generate the oil treatment as you keep busy around the house for an hour or so. You can also use an electric heating cap or sit under a bonnet dryer for about thirty or forty minutes.

When the time's up, remove the cap and reclip your hair into the sections. Before you wet your hair, apply a small dollop of shampoo to each section and then lather up with water. Shampoo only enough to remove oily residue from your hair.

If your hair is unprocessed, you can follow the hot-oil treatment with a moisturizing conditioner.

≋≋ De-Tangling

When de-tangling, always work from the ends of your hair, toward your scalp. If your hair is unprocessed, use a spritz of water on the section you're trying to unsnarl. Water is a natural softening agent and it works so well that I prefer to comb my hair only when it's dampened. You can also use a bit of creme rinse or moisturizing conditioner to help it along.

Combing

After you've de-tangled, part your hair into three or four sections with plastic clips. Undo a section, grab a handful of hair from the section, and pin the rest out of the way with the clip.

Use your wide-toothed comb and gently but firmly comb through the handful of hair. If you reach a snag, stop and use your fingers; don't try to pull the comb through.

As you de-tangle and comb each section, you can twist or pin it in a manner that will be easy for your braider to remove. If you're prepping your hair the night before a plaiting session, wrap your hair in a satin or silk scarf before you sleep. Your braider will probably re-section your hair to her own liking before braiding, but you will have made the job a little easier.

You'll find that if you wear your hair Afrocentrically or in styles that enhance coils and curls, you'll tend to use your fingers for everyday styling and the comb for parting or de-tangling. Fingers preserve more coils than combs do.

Shedding

If you remove snarls using your fingers rather than a comb, most or all of the hair that comes out will be shedded hair. Hair that has completed its growth cycle and been released from the follicle is shed. Hair that has been shed naturally has a whitened end from the dead root. If you're shedding an unusually large amount of hair, you should see a doctor.

Brushing

The point of brushing is to distribute scalp oils and brush away loose scales. If your hair is tightly coiled, you can't pull the brush through to the ends of the hair without tearing some of it out. Here's a smarter way to brush.

The Best Way to Brush. The best brush to use is a gentle, natural bristle brush. De-tangle your hair. Separate it into three or four sections for easier management if you like, but it's not necessary. Part your hair to the scalp and brush from the part, out to the ends.

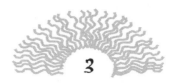

3

Who Ya Gonna Call?

As a former hair refugee, I occasionally suffer from nightmare flashbacks. Sometimes all it takes is hearing the word *touch-up* and I'm . . .

Back in the hair assembly line. Ebay has just rodded me up, but the phone rings and he hands me over to RaNeeva, who is supposed to be watching me under the dryer while my dry curl ("Waves today, natural-looking curls tomorrow") is processing, but she's also doing somebody else's precision cut and I know I wanted a dry curl, but is my hair supposed to feel this dry up under the plastic cap? Ebay yells back to RaNeeva about checking my curl. . . . "You feel dry?" asks RaNeeva without taking step one toward my dryer, and she tells Tetta to wet my rods with some more wave solution. I push the hood off my head and I sit and I wait while Tetta answers the phone on her way to get the wave solution. Then I push the plastic cap off the rollers and I wait . . . and the streetlights go on . . . and I wait . . . and still I wait . . . until I hear faint shouting from the back room and I reach up and touch my new-jack Brillo. I hear it again . . . sounds like . . . Tetta. "Neeva! We're out of the wave solution! Is the beauty supply still open?"

It's a really bad scene.

And so the idea of an Afrocentric salon sounded especially appealing to me. I envisioned a sort of hair nirvana, and I could hardly wait: lush plants, soothing roots music, pleasantly efficient sistas who wouldn't snatch you bald-headed just because your coils were on the tight side, tasty snacks to spell the hours of plaiting, the juiciest gossip—the Total Salon Experience.

As one natural hairstylist told me, "Women come to us because we don't do that other stuff. The regular salons really don't care about you not wanting the chemicals—they're going to do whatever they have to do to get the effect they think you want."

Many refugees like me are drawn to Afrocentric salons because they can push the right buttons, and after all, what's wrong with a little stroking and pampering? Isn't that supposed to be the nature of a salon?

But do not be misled; it may be a higher calling but it's still all about business. Some Afrocentric salons have a total follow-through on their philosophy. They require that their stylists have natural hair, and if one is hired with processed hair, she or he must grow it out as a condition of employment. It's about setting an example. But most stylists working in braiding salons are licensed cosmetologists, so they may offer standard services like "thermal texturizing"—press and curls, flatironing, or "hot work."

At other salons, the word *natural* may mean that their primary impetus is a chemical-free do, but if you lay your money down and say "please," the stylist *will* reach back and open up a jar of Bantu. Salons offering this service say that they do so because as "natural" people, they know the horrors of botched relaxers all too well, and if you must subject your head to this festering evil, let *them* do it for you—the *right* way.

In the state of New York, cosmetologists who work exclusively with unprocessed or natural black hair must obtain a special license to perform these services, which include braiding, wrapping, hair weaving, and locking. This means that some braiders are licensed *only* to perform braiding and related services, while others are trained in all areas of cosmetology. Braiders hope to get similar laws passed in other states. If you want to have your hair relaxed or receive chemical services in a braiding salon, it's in your interest to be sure the stylist is licensed to perform those services.

My purpose here is not to preach nappy-er than thou—I'm just observing the scene. Some ladies feel that an Afrocentric salon has no business backsliding into Eurocentric styling. But on the same note, a braiding salon shouldn't humiliate a client just because she has had an intimate and long-standing relationship with hair straighteners. What is important to you is the most important issue to consider.

If you're looking for braids, twists, and locks, it's best to seek out salons or stylists who earn 99.9 percent of their money performing those services. And for my money, it is also smart to bypass straight shops that "feature braiding" or "will do them on request." As the proprietor of one Afrocentric salon told me, "That's like going to Kentucky Fried Chicken and ordering a hamburger."

I once had the assumption that a braider's association with an established business implied a certain level of professionalism, quality, and consistency. After all, these were the sisters who declared that springy African hair would now and forever more reign supreme. No more waiting in hair assembly lines because of scheduling mistakes. Well, the lyrics have changed but the strains of an old, tired jam might creep through unless you know what to watch for.

How to Find Afrocentric Salons

You can check out the Yellow Pages, but the most foolproof method is to get in the streets and do the legwork. Ask ladies with great-looking hair where they got it done. You know what you like and how you want to look. Be courteous, be complimentary. Please don't be put off by women who get an attitude about you asking. Kindly excuse yourself and move on, but don't stop asking ladies until you get a line on where the action is. If the hair is looking especially fierce, be sure and get the name of the stylist. There is a hierarchy within each salon and some stylists are better than others. If the lady seems willing, you might ask about prices, but don't sweat it if she doesn't really want to say. What you're looking for is a ballpark figure because chances are pretty good that your head won't be priced the same, anyway. If you start to hear the same names more than once, you're probably onto something good. When you come up with two or three salons, you can begin lining up consultations.

Checking Out the Scene

In the straight world, unless you are dealing with top-notch stylists with extreme reputations behind them—say a John Atchison or an Olive Benson—routine consultations are pretty few and far between. More often than not, my request for a consultation was read as an affront to the stylist's professional expertise and the vibe was definitely "Make a hair appointment or go somewhere else." So you can understand my delight when I found that most Afrocentric salons encourage and even insist upon consultations.

Momentary euphoria aside, consultations simply make common sense when shopping for salon braids, twists, or locks. There's really no other way to assure yourself of a reasonably good rate of success. It is also a foolproof way to check out the vibe of the salon. Here are some factors to consider.

The setup. Do you have privacy or will you be on display? Personally, I don't care for being a living ad for the walk-in crowd at the mall. What if I fall asleep with my mouth open?

Would you mind spending a few hours in this place? Some of you will feel more comfortable in a formal setting where the current issues of *Ebony* and *Jet* are lined up, ready for your perusal, and a healthy stack of the past issues is within reach. Others will look forward to doing a little business with the brother selling jogging suits and kente hats.

What about food? If you're there for a marathon braiding session, is there a restaurant close by that will deliver, and if so, is there a place to eat in the salon?

Do you feel safe? Can folks just walk in off the street or must they be "buzzed" in to gain entry? (I'd feel better about an establishment that is selective about who walks through the door.) If you end up being there well after dark, will you need to arrange for an escort to your car? And just how is the parking situation, anyway? This is not trashing good salons that happen to be in areas that change character after dark, this is being sensible.

Here are some things that should make you consider taking your business somewhere else:

The receptionist who is also a consultant. I know that some salons try to offer this one, claiming that their stylists are too busy or "unavailable." Too busy to get paid, huh? This is doubly offensive when they have the nerve to charge money for the consultation. Trust me when I tell you, only a stylist can know for sure. So insist upon seeing one. I don't care if the receptionist has a doctorate of braiding—just say no.

Plenty of stylists and no receptionist. Someone has to answer the phone, make or break appointments, answer questions, and take messages. In all likelihood, if there is no designated receptionist, whoever answers the phone will forgo message taking and simply call the requested stylist to the phone, and it's probably going to be yours.

Stylists who seem to have telephone receivers attached to their heads and shoulders. I believe the only person who should have that sort of an appendage is the receptionist. At good salons, it's not too easy to get through to a stylist during working hours unless you're a close relation or it's an emergency. Too many frivolous calls and the salon soon has an opening for a new stylist.

Plenty of folks coolin' it in the waiting area. Tip: How to determine if this is a logjam of clients—discreetly ask a few how long they've been waiting and who they're waiting for. That should tell you all you need to know.

Consultations

Some salons charge a small fee for consultations—anywhere from ten to twenty-five dollars. Before I became familiar with salon protocol, I thought this sounded like a lot of money just to look at a style book. After I thought about it a bit more, the fee made good sense. If you put your money down, you are pretty well assured of a proper appointment and can expect a serious consultation. In turn, time is money for salons and they know your intentions are serious if you are willing to set up a paid consultation. The better salons will apply your consultation fee toward your first appointment, so you can both look upon the fee as an investment of goodwill. If you don't like the salon, at least you've only spent a fraction of what you would otherwise waste for a complete session.

If you aren't paying a fee or making a structured appointment for a consultation, you are running the risk of talking to the stylist while he or she is doing another head. I tend to get a little irritated when a stylist is trying to do justice to someone else when she is supposed to be doing my hair. And you, the prospective customer, are bound to feel as if you're intruding on someone else's time (and you are) if a stylist is trying to analyze your hair needs when she's in the middle of a cornrow.

Most consultations begin with a hair analysis. Because of this, most stylists would like to see you with your hair out or down, rather than up, so choose a style that you can reassemble fairly easily. During the hair analysis, the stylist will touch, stretch, and perhaps even wet a small section of your hair in order to determine its porosity, texture, and elasticity (ability to withstand stress). She should also ask you about your hair's chemical history, such as whether or not you've had any processing done, and if so, how long ago. This is not the time to start lying. The questions are necessary because a freshly relaxed head of hair may not be able to stand up to the tension of some braided styles, particularly extensions. In fact, if you're considering braided extension styles, it's not a good idea to have your hair relaxed or even touched up just for that purpose. This is one situation where your coily, natural hair will give you the styling advantage. If your hair tends to be especially dry or oily, or if you are plagued with an especially flaky scalp, now is the time to mention it.

The stylist will ask other questions, such as what kind of products you use, and how often you shampoo, condition, and lubricate your hair, and may recommend a product line he or she is familiar with. Usually, stylists will give you a brief overview of the services they provide. Somewhere during the consultation, you'll both get down to what it is you want and an estimate of how much it's going to cost you. This is the time to pay attention and speak up, frankly, about what you'd like. Most stylists will suggest you look at their book in order to become familiar with their salon style.

≋≋ How to Check Out a Style Book

The good thing about braids and twists is that you can actually bring in a photograph of, say, Janet Jackson à la *Poetic Justice* and leave the salon with a pretty reasonable facsimile. This is because literally anything is possible, depending upon the skill of the braider, the amount of time you want to spend, and your supply of cash. So we hone in on the skill factor, because when everything is said and done, it's all about the presentation. In the braiding world, most but not all of the time, price is an accurate indicator of what you're going to get. If it sounds too cheap to be true, it probably is.

So you've finally got the book in your hands. Notice where the photographs were taken and how recently. The salon may display magazine photographs on the walls or style board, but you *don't* want to see a style book full of magazine clips unless they are specifically credited to the salon. You *do* want to see real pictures of real clients. You should already have in mind what it is that you want. For example, if you want pencil-thin individuals, you should pay attention to the kind of individuals they do. Pay attention to the styling. If you want styles that can be considered professional, then a book full of flamboyant hip-hop styles may not be your cup of tea—but don't assume they can't do anything else. Ask the stylist. What you are trying to determine is the expertise of the stylists; do the styles look polished and professional, or do they look like $25 braid jobs?

When you see a style that appeals to you, please ask:

    ≋≋ What kind of style is it and which stylist did it?
    ≋≋ How long will it take?
    ≋≋ Does it require extensions?

≋ If so, what kind of extensions are required?
≋ Can it be done without extensions (if that's your pref-
  erence)?
≋ How long does it last?
≋ Can I shampoo it or does it require a "dry shampoo"?
≋ How much do you think it will cost?

Some Afrocentric salons promote the cultivation of unprocessed hair and will help you learn how to care for it between appointments. Get your money's worth—speak up, ask for the information. Again, don't become intimidated if you indeed have a perm and simply want to give your hair a respite before commencing with the lye. Most of these ladies have been there and they'll be happy to show you right. If you pick up on attitude, pick yourself up and leave. No hard feelings.

If you aren't too familiar with braids, locks, or twists, I suggest that you start slowly. If you are anything like I was, breathless at the possibility of leaving a salon with more hair than I ever dreamed of, you could become overwhelmed and make a bad first-time hair choice—like twelve-hour micro braids. Keep it simple and try to choose something that can be done in one or two hours. You can always come back for the big leagues later.

Time and Money

One thing to understand is that the nature of braiding is a little different from that of the straight world. Say you're on time for your appointment but your braider is working on a head with approximately three square inches of unbraided hair left. She's doing extensions and they're *individuals*. You're thinking, just like I was, Oh, she'll be done in about fifteen, twenty minutes. . . . Think again. To paraphrase Soulmaster Don Cornelius, "you can bet your bottom dollar" that you will be there at least another hour and probably more. Time is important when it comes to braids, locks, and twists. A stylist who not only can give realistic time estimates but deliver on them is a real find. When you see price lists that have a lot of hourly rates next to them, there's a good reason, and it's all about the ch-ching! of cash money.

Better salons will have prices posted somewhere obvious. I don't understand the logic behind not posting prices, although I do understand that in the case of Afrocentric styling, variables like the time it takes to braid, or the type or length of extension hair, often affect prices. Still, I think it is reasonable to be able to get a ballpark estimate as to how much services will cost. I believe most women today know that it is unrealistic to expect to get a good braid style for $40, but it is a real peeve to discover that those simple-looking cornrows are going to run you $350.

Salons cost more than freelancers. Prices change, so I'm not going to get into specifics, but this is pretty much the way it works.

$$$$
Micro braids, braid weaves, braid interlocks

$$$
Styles with extensions
Individuals
Goddess Braids
Casamas braids
Locks (starting locks, lock extensions)
Senegalese Twists
Styles using lin extensions

$$
Styles without extensions
Cornrows, twists, flat twists, braids
Thermal texturizing
Coloring

$
Trims, consultations, shampoo and conditioner

Here's an idea of how long you'll be in the chair and how long the style will last. (Styles using extensions take longer and last longer than styles without extensions. Braiders will suggest that you avoid wetting or shampooing styles braided without extensions.)

≋ Two or Three Months
Individuals with extensions, medium sized—four to six hours
Micro braids with extensions—twelve hours (sometimes
the time can be cut down if two braiders work simul-
taneously)
Lock extensions

≋ Two or Three Weeks
Goddess Braids—can take one or two hours, depending
upon the intricacy of the style
Individual twists without extensions—two to three hours
Flat twists—one and a half to two hours
Cornrows—depends on size and density

Freelancers

Having your hair done outside a traditional salon setting can be
a good experience if you choose wisely. In the best scenario, the
atmosphere is relaxed and casual. Also, with freelancers, you
have a good chance of being able to negotiate prices. But always
keep quality in mind, rather than the lowest prices, and you
should be able to get a satisfying freelance service.

I found a good freelance stylist through a referral from another
pleased customer, my friend Charmaine. Charmaine accompanied me to the stylist's home. The stylist gave me an informal
consultation at her home before I arranged to have my hair
twisted. What impressed me about "Imani" was the way she kept
her home—clean and fragrant with aromatic oils. She was a gra-
cious hostess and offered me a choice of fresh fruit juices. She
said she was about creating beauty through her work and I could
definitely get behind that. She had stacks of color photographs of
attractive, well-groomed clients—a casual style book.

Me being me, I kept asking her about exactly what it was she
did, so she told me to sit down and she'd show me. My hair was
not exactly fresh—in fact, it needed shampooing—so I tried to
ease my way out of it. Imani got out a chair. Time was running
out. I had worn my hair up because it really needed washing and
now I was about to be exposed. "Didn't you say you wanted to get

your locks twisted, Charmaine?" as I gave my friend the buck-eye. Girlfriend acted like she didn't know what I was talking about. "Girl, get in the chair." By then, Imani had a towel, hair fixins, and me in the chair, steadily making up excuses. She whipped out some cotton pads soaked in witch hazel and cleaned part of my scalp with them. "Yeah, you're right, it's a little flaky up in here— I'm going to rub a little of this Hair Booster on your scalp. You're going to feel a tingle. It's going to feel good. That's the cayenne in it." When she was done with that small section, it felt great. I wanted to run down to Sav-On and get an economy-sized bottle of that witch hazel and let her go for broke. When I left, I had an idea of her prices and the amount of time it would take to complete my individual twists (about two hours—but I added an extra hour to be sure). Imani asked if I'd like her to shampoo and condition my hair before twisting it, but I figured I'd save time (and face) by coming in with a clean head.

When the time came for the appointment, Imani was ready, with everything set up. I could smell something good cooking, and when I commented on it, she said she had on some greens and black-eyed peas warming up for me. They were delicious, well seasoned, and free of grease. "You don't need any hog to make your greens and beans taste good," Imani said. I heard that.

We talked about various things—hair, men, children, and more hair. While I was there, a couple of ladies came to see Imani but it was very cool, because she continued twisting me up and not a moment was lost. When one lady came with two children in tow, Imani told her she wouldn't be able to accommodate the children, but she could reschedule her appointment. She was polite but firm. The lady returned forty-five minutes later— alone. Imani welcomed her back and offered her a glass of juice.

I enjoyed chatting with her other customers about their locks and twists. Two hours later, Imani was done. The twists were even and uniform, and even though Imani suggested a trim, my hair looked great.

This was a very pleasurable experience and I was fortunate to find a braider/locktician who was professional in every sense of the word. They may not all serve a delicious lunch, but I think you have an idea of the kind of treatment to expect.

You can take the same steps to locate a freelancer that you would use to locate a good salon. Some freelancers have day jobs that limit their braiding time to evenings and weekends. Some freelance braiders provide services like shampoos and hot-oil treatments. In general, it's a good idea to come with clean, conditioned hair, ready for braiding.

A Good Braid Job

How do you know when you've been misled, hoodwinked, bamboozled? You've been played if:

≋The braid job was too cheap to be real. Deep down, you knew better but you just couldn't resist that bargain. There are exceptions, though—for example, children's hair should rate lower prices. Or, if there is a braid/lock price war going on, but even then, I'd just say no.

≋Your braids feel eye-popping tight, your scalp is stinging. The stylist tells you to use some braid spray and take some aspirin.

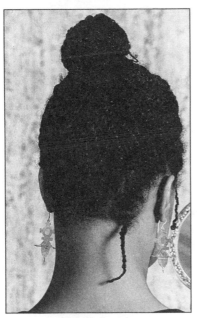

Variations on this include being advised to take "a scalp-relaxing shower." You know you've either been told to do this or know someone else who has. If the braids are that uncomfortable, the only thing that's going to give are the roots of your hairline. And once the roots are gone, they don't come back.

Two-strand twists sans extensions.

≋You leave the salon carrying the weight of the world on your shoulders. The base knots of your extensions can be seen from fifty yards away. These are signs that the braider used too much extension hair and that he or she is probably not very experienced. Heavy extensions can cause your own hair to pull out at the root. The style will loosen and parts will come undone. A good braider will be able to judge how much hair to use in each braid or cornrow, based on the texture and density of your own hair.

≋The price of your style is based on the amount of extension hair used—per package. Even if you're getting micro individuals or a braid weave designed to mimic straightened hair that requires a high quality of human hair, the extension hair should be figured into the total fee for the service. If you want to see an example of what can happen, check out the end of Chapter 10, "The Promised Land."

≋The salon charged you extra for braiding your hair to the ends. I once tried to save a few dollars in one of these salons. I was rewarded with an extremely unflattering, cornrowed extension style that was braided away from my hairline. The unbraided ends exploded into a stiff cascade on the back of my head, an effect my husband referred to as "The Rooster." Cock-a-Doodle-Do.

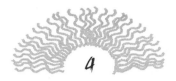

4

Every Braider Is a Star . . .
or knows One

Seems like every braider has a star story to tell. It must be exciting for braiders who actually do have celebrity clients. They must get to know them very well because when you spend five to seven hours in someone's hair, secrets are bound to come out. Or so I thought. In reality, the stylists with long-term celebrity clients are the ones who are smart enough to keep their mouths shut and their fingers moving. Or they put out just enough information so as not to offend the star clients, but keep people like me strung out so we come back for more stardust.

Name someone famous who has worn braids or locks—say, Ashford and Simpson or Peaches and Herb—and twenty stylists are going to have had an association with them. Some sister braiding on a beach in Jamaica is probably claiming this very minute that she took care of Bob Marley's locks when he was alive.

You've heard of Jerry's Kids? In Los Angeles, they've got Stevie's People. With all due respect to the braider or braiders who actually do Stevie Wonder's hair, because it must be a real trip to meet people coming and going who swear they are in His Circle. As soon as Stevie began wearing cornrows on a regular basis, half the braiders in L.A. claimed to have done them. Or else Stevie's people talked to them about doing him, but they wanted the braider to go through a bunch of changes and they didn't have time for that. I heard this one so many times it sounded like a tabloid headline: STEVIE WANTED MY SPECIAL TOUCH—BUT I HAD TO TURN HIM DOWN!

I was once informed by a man I met at a swap meet that the beads I was examining were in fact the same beads he had sold to Stevie.

"You mean . . . ?"

"That's right, my sista. Those cowries he had on for the Mandela concert? Those were mine."

"You mean Stevie Wonder came here? To the swap meet?"

"Sista. I didn't say *Stevie* came here, I said he was wearing my beads. His *people* handle that kind of stuff. Those are my best cowries, too, three dollars a package. But for you, my sista . . ." He looked around. "For you—four packs for nine."

When I got into braids, I was just as much into the star turn as the next customer. The fact that I was a college student on a limited budget but with an unlimited imagination probably just made me an easier sale. I knew plenty of folks who claimed to be kin or play cousin to some celebrity, anyhow.

That's why I loved going to Blossom's (whose name has been changed to protect her business) shop on Crenshaw to get my braids done. Blossom herself had that star quality about her—she was a dancer who happened to be taking a few courses at the university I attended. She herself was a walking advertisement for braids, she was lithe and attractive, and she sported small individuals pulled up into a thick ponytail.

Among the celebrities whom Blossom claimed as clients was none other than Bo Derek of *10* fame. Bo's hair was the talk of L.A., and the stylists who weren't saying they had braided her insisted she was wearing a wig. I wanted to know how her hair was really done, so I asked Blossom because she seemed to know it all. She didn't let me down.

"Oh, you didn't know?" Very casual, very cool. "*We* did her." My mouth dropped open as one of her braiders nodded a silent "Amen." Tell me more.

It took fourteen hours, she said, mostly because Bo's hair was very straight and the extensions tended to slip. So they anchored them down with a few stitches. They couldn't be washed or else they would slide right out, Blossom added.

"Slide right off her head," said another braider.

"Oh, you can braid white hair," Blossom said, "but you have to know how to do it or it will come right out. Bo's stylist went to the Braidin' Shack [name changed to protect that salon] first, then they came here"—and she paused for emphasis—"because *I know what I'm doing.*" I wasn't about to argue with that.

"Honey, some folks want what we've got, but they got to come back to the source. They've got to come—" She turned to her partner for testimony.

"Back to braids!" they both crowed.

I was just a tad suspicious. I'd seen the movie twice, just to check out Bo's hair. If she couldn't wash the braids, then what happened during the beach scenes, when she got wet? I asked Blossom.

"I had to do touch-ups," she said. "I have a day rate for clients on jobs like that." She lowered her voice meaningfully. "It costs a lot of money."

So it certainly didn't lower my opinion of Blossom's when I heard that none other than Darchelle from *Solid Gold* had her hair braided there.

Nowadays, folks snicker and roll their eyes at the mention of *Solid Gold*, but when it was first televised, the Solid Gold Dancers were the fly girls (and boys) of their day. The show featured Top 40 pop hits and chorus-line dance routines. *Solid Gold* was one of Hollywood's last attempts to cash in on the music market before videos took over.

Darchelle Wynn was probably the best advertising that Blossom's salon ever had. Everybody watched Darchelle fling it to and fro as a *Solid Gold* dancer each week. Her following and talent soon earned her a special credit as "Lead Dancer." The sista with the baddest body and the longest hair on the show. Darchelle, the extension queen.

There was a poster in Blossom's shop, of Darchelle doing the *Solid Gold* lunge, breasts and booty jutting out of her sequined spandex. Her trademark braids—individuals plaited small so they would appear to be a lush mane at first glance—trailed down her back and over her shoulders. That poster talked to me. It said, "Go ahead, child. Forget them bald-headed heifers. Get yourself some hair!"

First things first.

"*You* actually braided Darchelle's hair?"

Blossom worked it like any good businesswoman would in that situation.

"She was in here yesterday, girl. Just came back from taping the show. All that jumping around loosens those edges and she needed a touch-up," said Blossom as she scratched another part into my scalp.

"How does her hair really look?"

"About the same as yours," she said. So me and Darchelle had the same length of hair! I tried to crane my neck around to catch another look at the poster, but Blossom prodded my head back into position.

"She gets micro individuals. Takes about two days. I do a private session." This was a bit of a downer. I was getting one layer of budget-busting cornbraids for $125. Sure, I could do the braid down the back, the ponytail down the back, or wear it rolled in a bun at the nape of my neck, but that was about it. Versatile micros *started* at $500. Darchelle's were rumored to have cost more than $1,000. To me, this was Crazy Money, Big Money. But then, Darchelle was a big star with big hair needs. Hmmm, how much work-study money could I scrape together . . . $3.65 an hour, ten hours a week . . .

I'd just have to fake it with my cornbraids until I could get ahold of the cash. Meanwhile, who said I couldn't work on the body?

Several hours later, when Blossom was done, I walked out of the shop. Gigoloed my way to my Pinto with strains of "She's a Bad MamaJamma" going through my head. I had the hair. I was almost there.

One day a quiet woman in a fur coat was leaving the shop around the time I had come in to make an appointment. She had pretty milk chocolate skin and three layers of cornbraids. Blossom had stepped away to get something and the woman sat down near me. I asked her about her braids or something, and being nosy, I also asked what she did. She said she was a singer. Was she in a group or something? She said her name was Angela and that she was part of a duo, Rene and Angela. I wasn't familiar with their music, but I pretended that I was. It was a few years

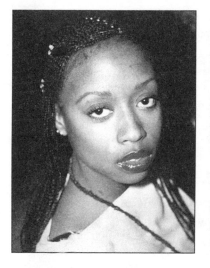 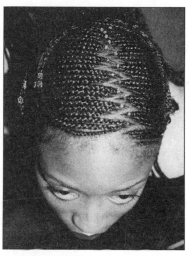

"She's a Bad MamaJamma" . . .
My *celebrity salon braids. Am I*
wearing enough lip gloss?

A bird's-eye view of my wanna-be
Solid Gold *cornbraids.*

later, after Angela Winbush had gone on to a successful solo career as a singer and songwriter, that I realized with whom I'd been chatting.

Then there was the woman who told me she had been one of Elvis's background singers. She was in to make an appointment. We chatted it up and she pointed to a gold pendant she was wearing that spelled out her name in diamonds. It was a gift from Elvis, she said. At the end of their gig, he had also given each singer a car, an El Dorado Cadillac. He was a nice man to work with and generous on top of it, she said. He was even nice to her mother.

"They say those things because they didn't know him," she said. "But Elvis knew how to treat his singers. They don't call him 'The King' for nothing, honey."

Then there was the matter of my wedding. I decided that since my husband-to-be and I were going to be honeymooning in the Bahamas that I should do something practical with my hair. I decided to get it braided. Then I could go buck wild in the surf and have no worries. Given my previous hair history, my folks kept their opinions to themselves when I told them I was to be married wearing braids. I thought they were being tactful. I realize now that they were probably rendered speechless.

So I hooked up with Maxine Jones. I got her number from an ad in an Oakland weekly. The ad was a replica of her business card, which had her picture on it and a phone number. Maxine Jones, Braid Artistry.

I arranged to meet Maxine in front of a salon in downtown Oakland. Her braiding studio was in a quiet nook on an upstairs floor. She was a little late for the consultation, but eventually she

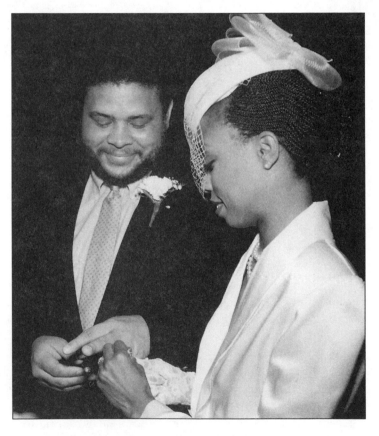

My "En Vogue" wedding . . . I remembered to get my hair braided, but forgot to "Hold On" to the wedding rings. With this college graduation ring, I thee wed . . .

appeared, driving up in a red BMW, a 320i, wearing small indi-viduals pulled up on top of her head. She was small in stature, but not bone thin, with light brown eyes. "Hi, I'm Maxine Jones," she said.

She did the consultation—I was getting two layers of shoulder-length cornbraids with extensions, an off-center part—and we set up the appointment. She had plenty of appointments already in her book, but I made one in plenty of time for the wedding. I checked out Maxine's own hair, and her individuals looked fresh and sharp. I asked who did her hair, and when she said that she did it herself, I was sold. Should I do anything special before she braided, like blow-drying or something? She said yeah, but that I shouldn't touch up my relaxer.

"When it comes to braiding," she said, "nappier is better." I've remembered that ever since.

Maxine had a very sweet manner and a soothing voice. She said she was from Paterson, New Jersey, but had come out to California to pursue a singing career. While she worked on me, during lulls in the conversation, she would hum and sing bits of songs in a pretty soprano. It was obvious that the girl was a con-tender. I asked what kind of singer she wanted to be, and she said she would love to get jobs singing jingles because a singer could make a good living doing that.

My do took about five hours. Maxine's work was good and I wore her braids for a couple of months after my wedding. The only thing was that I came back and wanted her to replace the second layer of cornbraids with individuals so I could pull them up, but she wouldn't do it. She said the top layer was too old and the whole head needed to be redone. That was the only way she'd do it. Of course, this involved more money than I could spend at the time. I was disappointed, but she was firm. Still, she was very sweet in her refusal.

So, when En Vogue exploded onto the scene and I saw that a member of the quartet was the same Maxine Jones who'd done my hair, I was surprised, to say the least. I checked out the first video, *Hold On*, so I could see Maxine's do. Sure enough, there she was sporting some micro individuals, braided small, in a shoulder-length cut. So much for those jingles.

Nowadays, if I mention that Maxine from En Vogue did my hair, folks aren't quite sure where I'm coming from. They probably think I'm just trying to be one of her people.

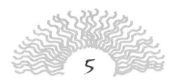

5

Yakety Yak

Some people remember things like the first time they saw Paris or Morocco. I remember the first time I saw extensions. It was spring semester and a new girl appeared at Vanden High. She wore cornrows that trailed past her shoulders. I admired them enviously, thinking to myself that it could have been me, if only my mother would cooperate. Then one day the sista strolled by wearing her real, short hair. I was flabbergasted.

"What happened to the sister's crop?" I asked my friend Milicent.

"What do you mean?"

"The braids—did she cut 'em or what?"

"Oh, that. Those were *extensions*, dummy."

Extensions? What the heck was she talking about?

"C'mon, she had braids. It was her hair. I saw it."

"Yeah, she wanted you to *think* it was her hair. It's like a weave. They just braid extra hair into your braids. Lon-neece," she said, shaking her head and laughing. "Where have you been?"

I'd been stuck in a time warp, begging in vain for lowly cornrows only to discover that a serious hair innovation had made the scene. Well, fancy that. As soon as I got out of Dodge, I was gonna get me some.

The very name given to the wefts of synthetic fibers and human and animal hair explains their purpose. Ancient Africans were using palm leaves, raffia, cotton, and wool to extend braided styles since before recorded history, and there is evidence that noblewomen in other parts of Africa passed on plaiting techniques to their Egyptian counterparts. The Senegalese are noted

masters of extension artistry and technique. In parts of Africa—
the Fulani of northern Nigeria, for example—extensions are
passed from mother to daughter, and a woman patronizing a
braider will use the family hair.

Today, extensions are a combination of aesthetic preference
and practicality. They can bridge the gap between what Mother
Nature neglected to provide and your idea of how you want to
look. For example, lin, a wool fiber, is commonly used to fill out
Goddess Braids and Senegalese Twists. Extensions can make
braided styles more durable so you're able to shampoo and swim
without washing out the plaits. Extensions can fill in a lot of
gaps, but your hair should be at least two inches long to provide
a proper anchor.

Are extensions mandatory? Depends upon who you ask. The
hair traders and manufacturers will almost certainly say yes. Folks
don't sit six hours or longer to get a style that will last all of two
weeks *without* extensions, say the jobbers. Your braider can complete a style in half the time if you skip the extensions, but it will
last only a maximum of two to three weeks, and that's *without*
shampooing. If you like to freshen your style more often than
every two or three months, nixing the extensions is a better
choice. The extensions themselves are only part of the equation;
it's the braider's skill *and* the quality of the extensions that determine whether you leave the chair with beautifully done braids or
with "nylon hair."

Back in the days of Peaches and Herb, braiders simply asked
what kind of hair you wanted, "human or synthetic?" "Ummm,
which is better?" "Human costs more but synthetic lasts longer,
unless you're getting individuals; then we use human."
Individuals were for the woman who wanted that long, flowing look achieved by braiding plaits so small that they almost
mimic straightened hair. They were also for the woman of
means. It stood to reason that if you were paying anywhere from
$500 to $1,500 for individuals, you might as well spring for the
human hair.

Nowadays, it's a different story. With styles ranging from cornrows to corkscrews, braiders use about four different types of
extensions—human, synthetic, fiber, and even animal hair. In
the United States, braiding salons usually have their own sources

for extension hair, which makes sense because they know which type of hair is necessary to achieve the effect the customer wants. If you're dealing with a reputable braiding salon, their hair source is going to be your best bet, unless you are extremely familiar with the hair trade.

If you patronize an independent or freelance braider, he or she will most likely tell you what kind of hair is required for the style you want. In the hair trade, there is such a thing as—dare I say this?—*good* hair. If you use extensions, you might as well aim for the best. Some freelance braiders have their own supplier; others will specify a certain type of hair and let you do the shopping. So let's shop.

Hair for Sale by Mail

The ads usually feature a sista with a whole lotta hair and some eye-catching copy. Here's one that caught my eye: "No Tangle! No Matt! No Friz Up! No Swell Up! [*sic*]." Or my personal favorite: "Hairs! Hairs! Hairs! 100 percent Human Hairs!! [*sic*]." One ad promised "cuticle free hair"—not what I would consider a desirable quality because once the cuticle is gone, the rest of the hair strand is on its way out. ("Cuticle free" refers to a method of minimizing tangling, but I'll tell you about that as we go on.)

These ads all promise great prices and they all swear they are the professionals' choice. "Four out of five weavers choose 100 percent human hairs!" Seriously, people, unless you are able to scoot on down to the "showroom" (and I say that with great "respect") and see the wares for yourself, I'd pass on the dicey-looking ads. It's simply too difficult for a novice to end up with a good color match and suitable texture. I know some of you live in places where you have no choice but to order by mail. For those people, I suggest checking out ads in cosmetological magazines like *Shoptalk*. Trade magazines cater to the salons, which, in turn, patronize hair suppliers. Before you put that check in the mail or give up the credit card number, call the supplier. Talk to someone in the showroom. Ask about free color swatches or hair samples before you buy. The better outfits will send you a free catalog. Most will even send you a book of stock and/or color samples—for a nominal fee, but it's well worth the money if you don't want to waste time with mistakes. In any case, please choose a company that has a guaranteed return/exchange policy.

The Wig Shop from Around the Way

Little Shop of Wigs, Wigworld, The Wig Wam, Wigstock, Hairfest—I've seen zillions of these shops, and yes, I've bought some of their hair. Don't act like I'm the only one. You can get a plastic sack o' hair for $3.99, but it will probably look and feel just like Barbie's. Ditto for the local beauty supply, except that you'll probably pay $5.99 and there will be less hair in the sack.

You may argue that all wig shops are not the same, that some of these establishments give good hair. This is true in some cases. One way to separate the wheat from the chaff is to simply notice what the shop is selling based on display. Are there plenty of wigs but the extension hair is in a dusty pile of plastic sacks in the back room or in a forgotten corner? The shops that do a lot of extension and weave business are going to have plenty of that type of hair available for your perusal, even if it's not in your actual reach.

If you live in a small town or an area where you ask about extensions and folks refer you to the telephone company, you may have to do more legwork. A wig shop is a good start. Ask if they do any custom wig work *on the premises*. Custom work requires a certain quality of human or synthetic hair stock. The shop could turn you on to some decent extension hair. You can also check with a beauty supply, but instead of buying that Barbie hair, ask the proprietor if he or she can order the good Barbie hair from a wholesaler.

The Hair Connection

These are the people who buy hair imported from Asia, India, South America, and other parts of the world and sell it to the wig shop around the way or other members of their trade. Don't be discouraged, because many will sell retail to the public. You'll get your best deals at the suppliers—don't look for dirt-cheap prices here, but you're going to see better hair and probably much more in the way of choices. Manufacturers are more apt to offer price breaks if you buy in quantity, simply because they are used to dealing with cosmetologists and hair shops that move a lot of hair.

It's easier to find manufacturers in the larger cities on the East and West Coasts, but that doesn't mean one couldn't be doing business in your town. When you scout the Yellow Pages, look for key words like "hair sold by the pound, wefted or in bulk," and companies that do custom wigs and hairpieces on the premises.

Most suppliers have showrooms with hair samples. The dealer will ask you what you want—hair for weaving, braiding, or extensions or hair in bulk. Weaving hair is sold in wefts; it is sewn into a curtain with a seam at the top called a weft. Hair for braiding and wig making is sold loose. Some hair is sold by weight, as in ounces or pounds, so have the information available before you make the trip. Unless you like living on the edge, it's always better to buy a little more than you think you'll need. There's nothing like that mad dash to the hair store, hiding under a scarf, hoping you won't run into anyone you know or would want to know.

Human Hair— The French Connection

If you want tiny micro braids or any style that leaves unbraided ends that you want to curl or wave, you'll probably be dealing with human hair. The names sound exotic—"French Refined!" "European Straight!" "Italian Mink!"—but just about all of it comes from Asia. The rest comes from India, South America, and parts of Europe. I am also pleased to announce we are now getting human hair of the nappy variety, known in the trade as "Imported Afro Hair." Hmmm. It would appear that virgin American Afro hair is not that easy to find anymore. Either that or "imported" sounds more expensive than "domestic."

The Ultimate Hair

One of the factors that creates tangles is the condition of the hair cuticle. It stands to reason that one package of hair could have been made up from more than one head of hair. Three different donors could have contributed to one pound of hair, and even though the grade may be #1 Acme, the strands could still reject one another and tangle. To minimize this possibility, the hair is laid so all the strands and their cuticles flow in the same direction. The manufacturers claim this is done painstakingly by hand. To ensure that the cuticle remains in the same direction, the hair is sold in wefts only. If you buy this hair and cut it off for braiding, the manufacturers say they can't guarantee that the hair won't tangle. This is very expensive hair, starting at around $170 for a quarter pound. Longer hair and lighter colors cost even more. All the dealers seem to offer it.

What you want is a decent grade of hair that isn't going to mat or tangle at the drop of a hat. That is why you want to deal with hair traders who know their business, otherwise you'll end up with the cheapie doll hair. But do remember that the hair is only going to look as good as you treat it. If you abuse the extension hair, even the $200 stuff is going to look bedraggled.

The names pretty much tell the story.

≋The Straight family: includes "PermStraight," "European Straight," and "Bone Straight." Straight textures are usually used for weaving. The textures will come wefted—sewn into hair curtains—or left loose in order to be used for the fusion techniques.

≋The Wave family: includes "Spanish Wave," "French Refined," "Deep Wave," "Wet and Wavy," "FullaWaves," whatever. This is where you get into your textures used for extensions as well as weaving, but the main attraction is the wave factor. You'll use the wave family for the individuals with ends left loose for crimping, curling, and spirals.

≋The Afro family: includes "Afro Kinky," "Imported Afro Hair," and "Jheri Curl." These textures involve synthetic hair that is treated to simulate these styles or human Afro hair.

Human hair is priced according to quality and length. Expect to pay at least $30 to $55 or more per quarter pound. The ads that refer to their product being "the best you can buy" or mention "cuticles" usually deal with hair that costs over $150 per quarter pound. Beware of the wig shop from around the way that has "100 percent human hair" on sale for $15. You're going to get what you pay for, and if it's ridiculously cheap, it may be cut with synthetic hair.

Synthetics and the Rest

This family includes the processed yak, unprocessed yak, lin or *laine*, and synthetics known by brand names like Kanekalon and Cornalon. Synthetics are also known as plastic nylon hair.

You'll deal in synthetics when you want hairstyles that require the finished plait ends to appear curved, as with Casamas braids, or styles like silky locks, where extension hair is wrapped around a braided extension and sealed. Sealing is usually done by burning the ends with a lighter and rolling the tips between the fingers. This can't be done with human hair extensions because the hair will simply ignite and burn until both the extension hair and your own hair are gone. Synthetic hair can also be dipped into hot water to make the extension more pliable or to shape the ends in styles like braided bobs into a blunt silhouette.

The Kanekalon and Cornalon brands are pretty reliable and you won't have a problem with the price, so I won't bother to get into them. Get the best that a reputable dealer recommends. I tried saving a few pennies on synthetic hair one time and ended up with a head full of cheap-looking nylon that itched for weeks, even after I soaked the hair in Flex as a last resort. I'd spent all that time and money to get hair past my shoulders, only to wear the braids up in a knot because my face and neck felt itchy every time the Barbie hair brushed against them.

There is a curious brand of hair I saw called Yakety, which was labeled as 100 percent human hair but marketed to have the property of processed yak hair. The yak is a bovine animal from Tibet that resembles a sort of hairy buffalo, and the hair from this animal resembles kinky hair. When the hair is processed, it resembles straightened Afro hair. All this for just $30! The texture reminded me of my own hair after it has been blown dry and pressed straight—silky, but limp and ready to go back at the suggestion of moisture. Why would someone want human hair with the property of animal hair and pay human hair prices for it? A hair trade sage answered the question like so: "Think about it—if it said 100 percent animal, who would buy it?"

When I asked about the allure of yak, most dealers said they didn't deal in the processed yak, but were quick to pull out some human hair that looked just like yak. They said that real yak tangles and mats too easily. One dealer whispered something about bogus dealers who sell human hair cut with yak. Another cautioned me about using real processed yak, saying that the chemicals used to process it tend to leach out onto the skin and scalp when the wearer sweats. Hey, the idea of using animal hair on my scalp is more distasteful than the thought of chemical seepage. And I daresay that there are sistas out there who would wear processed cat hair if it didn't revert and had that silky quality that they're lusting for. To each her own. The straightened yak or imitation human yak (if you're still with me here) is commonly used for weaving or extensions.

Now we get to the unprocessed yak. Nappy yak. It averages about $60 for a quarter pound of hair. Unprocessed yak can be used to simulate Nubian or African locked extensions. This is done by either palm-rolling loose hair into separate locks or braiding individual sections and frizzing the braids so that the braid pattern is obscured and it resembles locked hair. I must say that these could pass muster as real locks if you just couldn't wait to grow real ones, but I myself would just as soon wait. I've been told it takes anywhere from five to nine or even ten ounces to do an entire head, depending upon how your locks are fashioned. You can also buy yak precurled into tight corkscrew ringlets. Oh, yeah, these were *really* appealing. I could just see myself with a head full of these "ringlets," looking like a character in a low-budget biblical drama.

Next we have lin, also known as lyn or *laine* (French for wool). Lin is a woolen fiber processed until it is soft with a dull sheen. One dealer told me it was like horsehair. Makes you wanna run right out and get some, doesn't it? It can be sold in a roll, much like rolled medicinal cotton, or in packages. I've seen it priced at $25 for a two-and-a-half-pound package and $20 for a one-pound roll.

Lin is commonly used for Goddess Braids to give them that extra fullness and punch if your own hair isn't quite up to the job. It's also used in styles like Senegalese Twists, Corkscrews, and some flat twist styles, again to provide what nature has not. My question was, Can you shampoo your hair with this stuff braided up in it? Some dealers said no, dry wash only. Others told me you can, but you have to use a professional dryer because it tends to draw up, like fabric. The choice is yours.

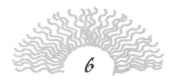

6

Stylin' and Profilin'

There are plenty of styles to choose from, but my purpose here is to show examples of some basic looks. You can check out hair magazines for the latest trends, and your braider and/or locktician can keep you abreast of things they can offer.

If you're considering styles that will work in professional settings, you'll want to keep it simple. Styles like cornrows, flat twists, Goddess Braids, or individuals that can be pulled into a sleek chignon or French (Nubian?) roll might work for you. Short, braided bobs are another option. Beads and other ornaments are not a good idea, and if you're addicted to length, I'd suggest that you choose styles that can be put up in a conservative manner. Long hair in a business setting can be distracting and unprofessional, whether it is braided or bone straight.

Locks are featured in the next chapter, "Lockin' It Up."

The following list is a compilation of basic braid techniques and styles.

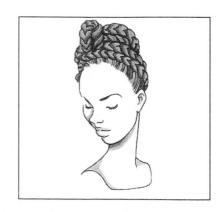

1. Goddess Braids. Usually done with lin extensions to pump up hair volume. If you need a conservative look, go for a less intricate pattern. Lasts up to two weeks.

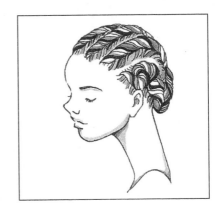

2. Flat twists or rolls. Hair is parted and twist rolled into patterns. Can be as elaborate or as simple as you like.

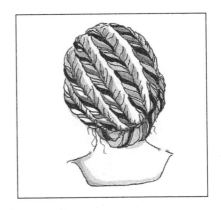

3. This is another look that can go to the office. Lasts up to two weeks.

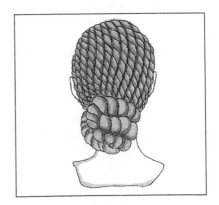

4. More flat twists. Think of these as two-strand cornrows. These can be done with or without lin (wool fiber) extensions. They'll last two weeks.

5. Individual
Senegalese braids.
The ends are tapered to
give the look of real hair.
Synthetic extensions will
help these last for two or
three months.

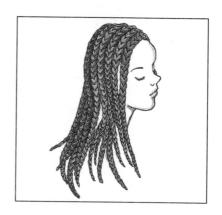

6. Individual two-
strand Senegalese Twists.
These are done using syn-
thetic hair extensions or
lin. Lasts for three months.

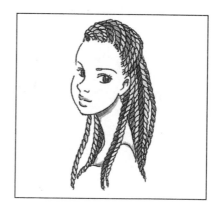

7. Corkscrews.
These can be done using
lin or synthetic extensions.
Can last two months.

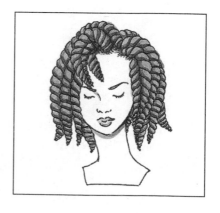

≋ How Corkscrews Are Done

The lin extension is
attached to the base
of hair section so it hangs
like a loose tail. Then
thread or cord is wrapped
around the tail until
it looks like this . . .

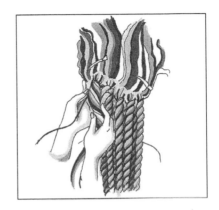

. . . or this.

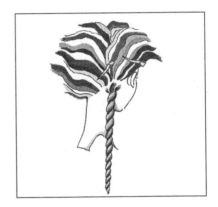

The string is pushed up
from the bottom until it
puffs into a corkscrew.

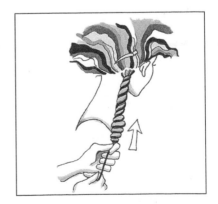

8. Cornrows.
The classic standby. If you use extensions, they can last for two months. Without them, they'll last about two weeks.

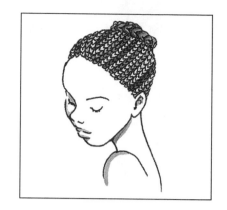

9. Bobbed individuals.
The curved shape can be achieved by a braiding method called stitching, which creates tension in the ends of the braids and curves them. Synthetic extensions are often burned and softened in hot water. The ends can also be "bumped" with a curling iron.

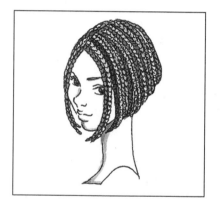

10. Cornbraids.
The hair is cornrowed and the ends are braided to hang free. This style can be done in layers for added thickness.

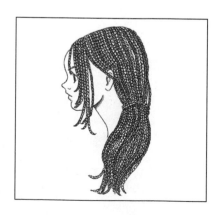

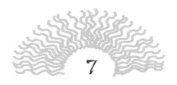

7

Lockin' It Up

Natty dreads. Dreadlocks. Cultivated locks. Nubian locks. African locks. A head full of short coils, gleaming in the sunlight. Thick horns of natty dreads. Long locks pulled up into a thick roll or bun. Plaited locks. A coiled bob.

A most impressive sight is a woman with beautifully groomed, waist-length locks. It is an extremely attractive look. Black women who are able to wear long locks turn as many heads as women with naturally straight hair of the same length.

If the Afro was the cutting edge in African hair during the 1960s then locks are the Afro of the 90s. The Afro was an American interpretation of the cropped, African coiffure. When it returned to the basic, cropped shape, it endured as a classic hairstyle for a woman of African descent with tightly coiled hair.

Locks do more signifying than an Afro or braids ever did. They signify uncompromised African hair. Like the Afro, they've had a rocky start. Locks put a different slant on the whole "hair question," if, in fact, there should even be one. Many people assume that locks are worn for political or spiritual reasons, and this may be true for some people, but most wear them simply because they like them.

The cropped natural evolved into a classic, and locks will become a classic alternative as well. Locks are a hairdressing option, just like a cropped natural, braids, cornrows, twists, or any other style.

Like the Afro, locks have been around in various forms for a long, long time. The Himba women in Namibia twist their hair with sheep's wool and coat it with a mixture of mud, fat, and ochre, a claylike iron oxide with a reddish tinge. The result resembles locks. The Samburu men of Northwest Kenya sport braids coated with red or yellow ochre, while the women wear their hair closely shaved. Wearing elaborate plaits protected and adorned with various coatings like ochre and animal fat is a widespread and ancient practice in African societies. The men of the Masai tribe of Kenya coat thin braids with ochre and animal fat, and wear soft leather caps to protect their hair while they sleep. Masai women keep their heads closely shaved, the better to show off jewelry. The men of the Kenyan Pokot tribe encourage their hair to lock into a large, flat mudpack bun, which they call Ancestor Hair. The bun often reaches down to their waists. Pokot women may shave their heads and braid the crown in tiny plaits. Turkana women wear finely braided locks with the sides or back of their heads shaved.

Locks will continue all over the Diaspora in one form or another, simply because they encourage maximum growth of tightly coiled hair in a lush manner. Why do you think so many women want to know how to grow them?

Dreadlocks. The Rastafarians say that they are named for the dread they hope to inspire with them, so they encourage their locks to merge together unevenly, until some look like great matted horns shooting from their heads. Another explanation is that dreadlocks came from slave traders who referred to the hair of newly arrived African slaves as "dreadful locks." The slave traders hadn't thought about how their own hair would look after months of lying in filth in the hold of a slave ship.

African or Nubian locks. These are the meticulously groomed locks that most African-Americans who wear them favor. The locks can be shaped, colored, layered, blunt-cut, plaited—they can be worked into many looks.

I first saw locks in the early eighties on the late actress Rosalind Cash while attending a Dance Theatre of Harlem performance in Pasadena. Being young, I noticed her glamorous fur coat first, then I noticed her hair. To me, it appeared to be in a halo of coils that was midlength between her chin and shoulders. I had no idea what style it was, but after making inquiries, I discovered that Ms. Cash was locking her hair. Oh, *that's* how you get dreadlocks, I thought. I had seen another actress at the same event whose hair was straightened in a pageboy that moved in the breeze, but it was Ms. Cash who made the biggest impression on me.

As time passed, I'd see Ms. Cash in various productions, and her hair flowed past her shoulders and down her back, while I passed through jheri curls, hot-combing, relaxers, and back again, wondering why my hair wasn't growing. And I've seen this happen time and time again with other women who have locked hair. Their hair flourishes.

Locks are a style that shows the coiled nature of African hair to its utmost advantage. Unlike braiding and straightening, locking the hair maximizes its growth to the point where it is common to see women with tightly coiled hair that is shoulder and waist length, women who could not achieve the same results if their hair was straightened.

Anatomy of a Lock: A Matter of Aesthetics

Hair grows for about three years before it goes into a resting phase and is shed from the follicle. Tightly coiled hair appears to grow more slowly because curl contracts the true length of the hair strand, but rest assured that African hair grows like any other hair texture. A three-year-old hair strand, under the best conditions, should be about twenty-four inches long, or almost waist length. Of course, length will vary due to factors like hereditary growth and curl patterns—tightly coiled hair, for instance, will appear to be shorter because of the spring factor. But those who covet long hair will be very happy with even half the average length. Remember, though, that the growth process is usually compromised by the insidious breakage that can occur as a result of sleeping on rollers, too much blow-drying, hot-combing, or chemical straightening. Out of all the styles for tightly coiled hair, locks have the potential for this kind of length.

When coiled hair grows undisturbed, the strands entwine around one another and cluster into random patterns. Shampooing or wetting the hair encourages these clusters to tighten, and if the hair is left undisturbed, except for shampooing or oiling, it will continue to grow. The hairs that are shed remain in the cluster and it appears to be matted. After a certain point, the cluster cannot be combed through or untangled—the hair is "locked." This is the process that occurs with Rastafarian dreadlocks, or uncultivated locks.

With cultivated locks, the size and pattern of each cluster of coils is determined by twisting, comb rolling, or palm rolling. This is how some people with locks achieve uniformly formed locked coils. The appearance of locks depends on your hereditary curl pattern and how your locks are started—that is, whether they are cultivated or randomly formed.

Who Do You Call?

There is more than one way to start the locking process. The ideal situation is to have a locktician or braider start your locks for you. A locktician is an Afrocentric stylist who specializes in starting and styling locks. You can find a locktician in the same manner you would find any other Afrocentric stylist or salon (see Chapter 3, "Who Ya Gonna Call?"). If a stylist isn't conveniently located, you could arrange a session to start them off and then follow his or her instructions on how to maintain them. If you have any weak moments in deciding about whether or not to wear locks, a visit to a good locktician can do miracles for your self-esteem. Lockticians give you positive reinforcement about wearing and caring for locks, plus a great-looking head of hair. You'll meet other people who admire and wear this hairstyle, and can share lock tales and grooming tips. You can, of course, start and groom your own locks, but get a friend to help with the initial partings so your locks will appear evenly formed.

Preparing to Lock

Start with hair that has been shampooed and conditioned, preferably with a hot-oil treatment. You can prepare your hair for locking in the same manner you would for braiding or twisting.

The one requirement that knocks a lot of people out of the game is that in order to do locks the hair must be *au naturel*. No chemical straighteners, no curly perms. Just you. Some people only want long locks, and when they discover that they'll have to cut off the perm, they fall off to the wayside.

Some people want locks but are afraid of looking like Buckwheat until their hair grows out. I had the same feelings when I cut my hair short and began wearing short twists while it was growing out. As I learned how to style and groom my hair, though, I felt better about it. There is an adjustment period that you and your hair will go through and I'll discuss some ways to deal with it, but before we get there, let's talk about the other requirement, perseverance.

It takes about six to eight months to get your hair to the point where it is recognizable as locked. This is an average estimate—it depends upon your natural curl pattern, as tightly coiled hair locks faster than loosely coiled hair. For some people, six to eight months is too long; they want some locks to throw over their shoulders by next week. There are also people like me who love locks, but know good and well that by this time next year, they'll want cornrows, twists, or something else. Once your hair is locked, you have to start from ground zero if you want to change to something else. Wearing coils is a good way to feed lock hunger if you aren't ready for a hair commitment.

Let's clear up a common rumor about starting locks. Folks get to whispering about beeswax, lemon juice, beer and vinegar rinses, glue—whatever. If your natural hair texture is tightly coiled or extremely curly, you don't need any of that stuff. Attempting to lock hair that is naturally straight or loosely waved, though, is difficult and often impossible, but people have used things like wax and glue to try and make it work. They end up with "matlocks," and trust me, you probably won't find it very

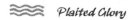

appealing. Locking these textures is like making extremely coiled hair bone straight—it can be done, but it won't be easy and it may be more trouble than the hair can stand.

≋ The Tools You Need to Start

Water in a spray bottle for dampening your hair and encouraging it to coil. You can also use leave-in conditioner in a spray formula or make your own herbal infusion. Many lockticians have their own special formulas. You can try rosemary and nettle, steeped in four cups of water. You can buy the dried herbs at health food stores, or find branches of fresh rosemary in your supermarket produce section and the dried herb where the spices are kept.

Plastic clips to separate your hair into sections.

Mirrors so you can see what you're doing from all angles.

A friend to help you if you aren't good with the mirrors.

A holding agent like a pomade or setting gel is optional. They help if your hair is loosely curled or you reach a resistant area. The idea is to help hold the locks in position until the hair relaxes into the coiled pattern. A water-soluble holding agent can be washed away easily without leaving a sticky film, which is why beeswax is not recommended. It might get you started, but you'll probably unravel your new locks trying to remove the residue from your hair.

A bonnet-style hair dryer will help set holding agents like setting gels and pomades. You can also let your newly twisted locks dry naturally if you see that your hair forms tight coils easily.

Locking Short Hair

Note: If you are starting your own short locks, draft a friend to help you.

≋ Braiding

Part your hair in sections about the width of your finger and braid each section into small plaits. If your hair is very loosely curled, you can apply a styling gel or pomade like Nu-Nile, Dax, or Royal Crown to help hold the plait together. Part the hair in the manner in which you'd like your locks to fall.

≋ Comb or Finger Twisting

You'll need a fine-toothed comb and a friend to help you with this method. Begin at your neckline. Use clips to separate the uncoiled hair from the coils. Take sections about the width of a finger or one half inch. Dampen the section with spritz and holding gel. Insert the comb at the end of the section and use it to twist the hair until it forms a coil.

You can also form small coils by twisting the sections between your fingers. Again, it is best if a friend helps you out.

Style Note: Coils are very chic, especially when the hair is short, and can be worn even if you don't plan to permanently lock your hair. They'll last at least two weeks before you'll feel the urge to shampoo. Just tie them up at night with a satin or tightly woven silk scarf.

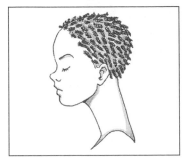

Coils or baby locks can be worn as a temporary style or the means to starting long locks. They can be palm-rolled or comb-twisted.

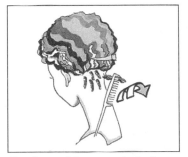

For the comb/twist method, dampen a half-inch section or a section about the width of your finger. Insert a small-toothed comb at the end of the section and twist the hair until it coils.

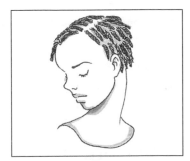

Longer palm-rolled locks.

Locking Hair
That's Mid-length or Longer

≈≈≈ Palm Rolling

Starting from the nape of your neck, take sections of the hair, about the width of a finger. If the section is too small, the lock will thin out and break off. Dampen the section with water or leave-in conditioner. If your hair responds to gel, use a bit of that, too. Roll the section between your palms, encouraging the hair to roll into a cylindrical coil or tight spiral. Continue rolling until all your hair is coiled.

≈≈≈ Two-Strand Twists

Starting from the nape of your neck, take sections of your hair, no more than an inch wide. Dampen the section with water and/or your holding agent and separate it into two strands. Twist the strands together in a ropelike manner, as if you were doing braid-style twists. The ends will coil around one another, and if they want to unfurl, give them an extra spritz of water and retwist them.

How to Care for Your Locks

The hardest part of grooming locks is getting through the transition period. After your locks are twisted, you must avoid shampooing for at least a month, in order to establish the coiling pattern. I went for almost four weeks without shampooing my twists before I finally caved in. You can probably gut it out for at least that long. If you shampoo any earlier, you'll probably end up with a natural or, at the least, with a whole lot of locks to retwist.

≈≈≈ Cleaning Your Scalp During the First Weeks

First, be sure and cover your locks with a scarf before sleeping. This will keep them neat and clean until your first shampoo. You'll also want to cover them for sleeping because it protects your hair no matter what style you're wearing.

Moisten a cotton pad or swab with an antiseptic skin cleanser.

Swab or clean the scalp exposed by the partings. I've used Sea Breeze or similar products. You can also use products like Listerine or witch hazel, although witch hazel is a mild skin toner and is better if you only need a light cleaning. The antiseptic skin cleansers are designed to lift grime, and that's what you want removed from your scalp. You can also run antiseptic-dampened cotton pads over the locks themselves to freshen them up.

If you make a habit of cleaning your scalp each week, you'll be able to minimize any itching you might have. If you wait until your scalp starts itching, like I did with my twists, you'll probably end up washing your hair after a week. If you do, just retwist your hair.

Finish the cleansing with a light oil if your hair tends to be dry, and retwist new growth and locks that have unfurled.

Be prepared for the fact that some people have not been exposed to tightly coiled hair in a style that accentuates this asset. Some of these people will have hair that is tighter than yours. They will probably dismiss your hair with the usual tired comments. For a morale boost, check out Chapter 8, "Surviving the Nap Patrol."

≋ Preening Your Locks

Locks are a style that looks best when the hair is "rich." A lot of women notice that their hair is more manageable when it isn't squeaky clean, after hair oils have had a chance to make the hair supple but before they have been weighted down with dirt. This is the state you want to encourage with locked hair. Therefore, most experts recommend shampooing every two weeks. Three is even better. If you want to shampoo more often, do so, but you must lubricate your locks to keep them supple between shampoos. You can use hot-oil treatments just as you would with braids, twists, or a cropped Afro.

≋ Shampooing

If you have long locks, it's easier to shampoo if you separate them into three or four sections with plastic clips before you start.

Wash your hair in the shower; a removable shower attachment

makes rinsing easier. As in shampooing braids or extensions, you want to concentrate on cleansing your scalp first, then smoothing the lather down the length of each section of locks. Squeeze the shampoo through the length of the locks and rinse thoroughly. Rinsing each section for two or three minutes is a good idea, because you want to make sure to remove all traces of soap from your locks.

If your locks are shorter and you've had a hard time keeping them twisted, you can try working shampoo into them and protecting the coils with a stocking cap during the rinse. The stocking cap is made using a *stocking*, not panty hose. Cut off the stocking at midthigh and knot the end opposite from the band to form a cap.

≋≋ Conditioning

The best type of conditioner to use is a leave-in formula, with a watery, fluid consistency, because it is less likely to leave a visible residue on your locks. You can also use moisturizing conditioners, but you must make a special effort to rinse them out or you'll have gummy locks. As long as you avoid excessive blow-drying, the main requirements for maintaining your locks are moisturizing and lubrication. Locks thrive on regular hot-oil treatments, and you can use the same techniques that are suggested in Chapter 2, "Four Degrees of Preparation."

Adjusting to Your New Look

The other hard part about locks involves maintaining a strong character. If you are used to wearing styles that accentuate tightly coiled hair, then it won't be too much of a long stretch for you to start locks. When you first begin locking, your hair will be in a tight coil stage. Depending upon how diligently you keep them groomed, you should have a head of tight little coils. I think this is extremely chic and pretty. As your hair grows, the roots will curl and the ends will coil. Some textures will resemble a coiled-up natural and others will separate into little rolled springs. Some days your hair will be really cute. Other days, you'll need a little help. Here are a couple of suggestions:

≋≋ Hair isn't cooperating today? Wrap a pretty scarf around your hairline and let the coils frame the scarf.

≋≋ Don't pack your hair down in an effort to make the coils less "Buckwheatish." It's okay to shape them into an even halo, but packing crushes your budding locks and it looks un-flattering.

≋≋ Make time to retwist your locks or you'll have more naps and frizziness than coils. Keep your hair lubricated; supple hair makes better coils.

≋≋ Meet other women who wear locks. Ask them how they started theirs and what it was like. If you meet a woman who doesn't want to talk about it, excuse yourself and move on. There are others who will be glad to discuss it.

≋≋ Don't become discouraged and get lazy about keeping up with your locks. This is a temporary growth stage and it will soon pass.

Lock Extensions

There are two schools of thought regarding lock extensions. Some lockticians will suggest lock alternatives for people who say they want locks but don't want to wait several months to estab-lish them. In this case, extensions are used as a starting point, and when the hair has reached the locking stage, the extension is removed. Extensions can also be used to fill out thin locks or extend the length of natural locks, or for those with naturally straight or loosely curled hair that resists locking.

Others don't believe in lock extensions. They say that locks are more than a hair fashion and those who aren't willing to culti-vate them naturally aren't ready to wear them. They say lock extensions are a temporary style that must be removed when their time is up and they aren't as appealing as naturally culti-vated locks. They also warn against using lock extensions as a transition to real locks, because your own hair can fuse or mat onto the extension and then the extension must be removed along with your hair.

I'm not about to step into *that* puddle. Why and how you choose to lock are up to you. If you're considering lock extensions, it's best to consult a locktician or Afrocentric stylist. Examine different extension methods and draw your own conclusions.

Each stylist has his or her own name for the extension method they like to use, and many times there are three different names for the same method. I'll use a simple description for each method of extension (most of these methods are adaptations of African thread wrapping, which is also called threading).

≋ Silky Locks

The hair is braided into individual extensions. Each extension is wrapped with synthetic hair, as in the African threading technique. The braid is wrapped from the extension base knot to the tip. The ends are sealed by burning and rolling them between the fingers. The result is a shiny-looking lock. Stylists sometimes get creative with this one, alternating different shades of wrapping hair on the same braid, forming ringed patterns. Instead of the matte appearance of naturally locked hair, Silky Locks have a distinctive shine. They attempt to simulate perfectly coiled hair that has not matted into locks, but no one will mistake these for the real thing. They'll last for about three months.

≋ Lock Fusion

The hair is parted into sections for locking. The sections can be prepared by palm rolling, twisting, or micro braiding. Extensions of human Afro hair are braided and the braid pattern is roughened with a stiff brush to obscure the braid pattern. The frizzed braid is palm-rolled to simulate a coil of locked hair. Palm-rolling the braid results in the matte look of natural locks. The lock extensions are fused

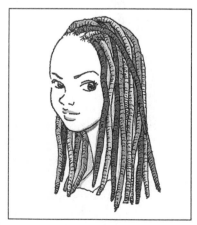

An American interpretation of African hair-wrapping and -threading techniques.

to the sections of natural hair using the same method used for bond weaves, with a modified hot-glue gun and pellets of hair-bonding wax. The look is much more realistic than other extension methods and has been used as a permanent lock replacement or transition tool. If you use lock fusion as a temporary extension, they'll last about three months.

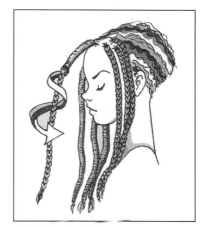

Individual braid extensions are wrapped with synthetic extension hair. The ends are sealed by burning the ends and rolling the softened tips between the fingers.

≈≈≈ Yarn Locks

The hair is braided into individual extensions. Each braid is wrapped with a single-ply yarn from root to end, as in the African thread wrap method. The ends are burned and rolled. The yarn gives each lock a matte finish that isn't as obvious as Silky Locks. If the yarn shade matches the hair color, it can be a conservative lock alternative. Again, you can get creative with this one, using different colors of yarn. Yarn locks can be shampooed like most other extensions. Use a satin scarf to cover yarn locks at night, to cut down on lint. They should last for three months.

≈≈≈ Yarn Braid Locks

The hair is braided into individuals that use strands of single-ply yarn. The ends are burned and rolled. The yarn cuts the shine on the synthetic extension hair, giving it a braid-lock effect.

≈≈≈ Maintaining Lock Extensions

Most stylists recommend a two- or three-week delay before the first shampoo. After that, it's okay to go ahead and use mild shampoo and leave-in conditioners. These styles—except for human-hair lock fusion—will take a bit longer to dry than natural locks, because of the layers of extensions (remember, the braid extension is covered by the wrapped extension).

Free Your Mind and Your Locks Will Flourish

People may assume that you're wearing locks because you're a Rastafarian or have a certain lifestyle or set of beliefs, but there are just as many people who wear them simply because they like them and like the way they look.

I like them because they look good, and they say, "You can have tight—okay, nappy—coiled hair that is long and lush." A lot of women grow locks because they want long hair. After they see that growing the hair is no problem, they cut the locks into different styles and sometimes even cut them off completely and start all over again.

Some women kind of slide into locks by experimenting with twists and small braids to see how they look. That's how Connie Melton began hers. Connie, who describes herself as "a long-haired girl," wore perms but always liked Afrocentric styles. A good friend of hers began wearing locks and that gave Connie the final push. She twisted her hair and then "just let the twists kind of take over." She'd shampoo, and some of the locks would come out, and she'd just retwist them until they began to stay that way. You can see the results of Connie's method in the photograph. She is a pretty woman to begin with, but the locks really make her beauty stand out.

When she first started her locks, Connie didn't know too much about the process, other than letting the hair coil. So whenever she saw someone else wearing them, she'd ask how they took care of them. Connie expected them to be as excited as she was, so she was surprised when some of them fronted on her.

"I assumed [it] would be kind of a secret society, but I didn't expect it to keep *me* out. I remember seeing a lady with perfect locks. They were all perfectly shaped—about the size of a pipe cleaner. She claimed she only washed them and kinda fluffed them out." Hmmm, sounds like a member of the secret society of lock perpetrators . . .

Capril Bonner-Thomas started locks because they complement her sense of style.

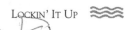

"I just wanted to be myself," she said.

It wasn't about having long hair, because this is a woman who has never had a hair deficiency. Her hair is abundant and full of springy coils. She is another example of a pretty woman whose locks have highlighted her beauty. People constantly compliment her style.

Capril's locks were started by a locktician, using the palm-roll and twist methods. It took about three months for her coils to lock. Once they began to "drop," or show length, grooming became a lot

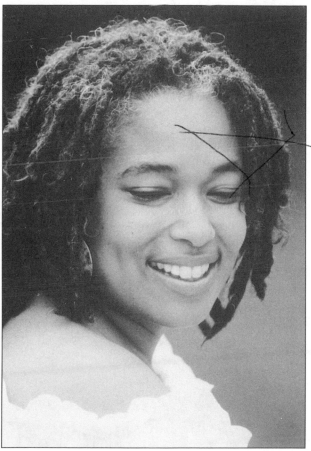

Not bad locks for someone who "just kinda figured it out."
Wish I knew how to stumble like that . . .

93

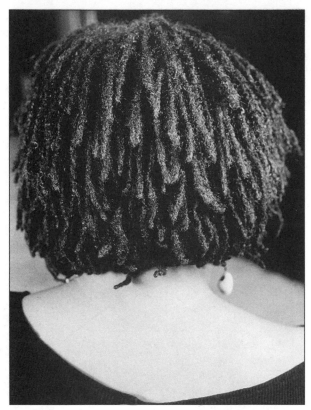

Good hair means never having to worry about the back view.

easier. Her locks are about a year old in this photograph. She exercises regularly several times a week and works up a sweat, so she freshens her hair with an after-workout rinse. She shampoos whenever her hair needs it, which is usually once a week.

Your Career as a Hair Ambassador . . .

Can't beat around the bush on this one. Some people associate locks with being nasty and unkempt, and they'll try to put you into the same bag. Think back to the sixties when the natural received the same "crime against cleanliness" rap. Nowadays, some of these same people will tell you that they'd rather see you with a natural than with locks. Go figure. What you can do is control how you present yourself. The women I see wearing locks are some chic, well-groomed ladies. Follow their example.

Above all, keep your head up. Enjoy your hair. Life is too short.

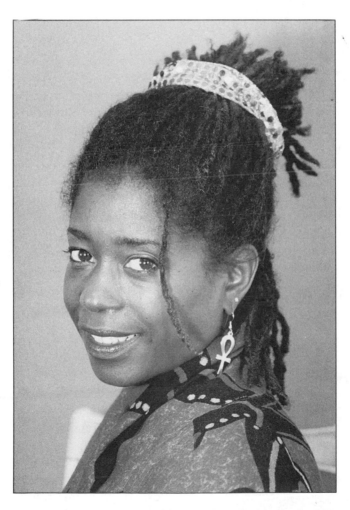

Queen Raziya—a master locktician with the locks to back it up.

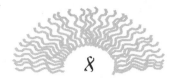

Surviving the Nap Patrol

Afrocentric styles showcase another facet of beauty. You will attract a lot of admiration when you wear them. Many women have told me that since they began wearing their hair in an Afrocentric manner that is becoming to them, they have been complimented at a rate that seldom occurred when their hair was straightened. This is not a criticism of straightened hair; it is simply an observation. Perhaps chemical straightening wasn't suitable to their hair texture, but they struggled to maintain it or they chose a straightened look that wasn't flattering. The same rules apply for Afrocentric styles; some will suit you better than others.

You will also attract attention from the Nap Patrol. Members of the Nap Patrol are people who make it their business to make you feel bad about your hair. Patrollers have been around in various guises throughout the black Diaspora since folks with coiled hair were first dispersed. The Nap Patrol enjoyed a resurgence in this country when the natural was introduced. Since then, Afrocentric styles have remained in favor, and this has caused many retirees to saddle up for another skirmish.

Some of these people suffer from Nappy Hair Phobia. They think their own tightly coiled hair is ugly and they want you to feel ugly, too. Others may simply view unstraightened hair as being less fashionable than straightened styles and refuse to practice the common courtesy of keeping their opinions to themselves.

Some black people have almost exactly the same response to locks and braids as they did to Afros in the 1960s. Back then, there were actually reports of people shedding tears over the sight of a woman wearing a natural. (A lot of these tears were probably shed during holidays and family gatherings when mothers tearfully apologized for photos ruined by the image of their child's Afro.) Ministers preached sermons against the Afro. Hairdressers claimed naturals were unsanitary and that straightening the hair kept it clean. Black women were often the most hostile, as if the act of not straightening the hair exposed a closely guarded racial secret. The best way to deal with the Nap Patrol is to continue to enjoy your hair and keep it looking fierce. Here are some suggestions on dealing with those negative vibes.

≋ When a Nap Patroller is bugging you about your hair, don't allow her to hurt your feelings or make you angry. Listen to her (if you don't have anything better to do). It's probably hard for her to see your pretty braids, long locks, or chic natural, knowing she's about to spend another sleepless night in sponge rollers. She may be cranky because she had an accident with the curling iron that morning. Picture her on a rainy day, desperately trying to make a hat out of newspaper because another Patroller stole her umbrella. Try not to laugh in front of the Patroller.

≋ Have professional photographs taken. Try a glamour shot or something provocative.

≋ Think about how full and healthy your hair will be due to your braids or twists.

≋ Take swimming lessons if you can't swim. Go to the beach and get into the water.

≋ Use the sauna room at your health club.

≋ Ride in a friend's convertible with the top down.

I'll Work for Food and a Home Relaxer kit

Substitute "locks" for "Afro" and it's déjà vu. It's reached the point where some folks are afraid of hair that even vaguely resembles locks. A friend related her experience of wearing her hair in twists. After unfurling them so they resembled crimped corkscrews, she encountered a relative who had heard about her hairstyle. This relative addressed—rather, accosted—my friend in the tone one would use to address a criminal.

"You *are* wearing DREADLOCKS!" she said, and turned to her husband. "I *told* you those were dreadlocks!"

My favorite is the teacher who had the audacity to send a note home to a child's mother, asking her to get the child's hair "done."

People will also justify their insults by claiming that "it's only for your own good," or that they're concerned about your employment/marriage/education/health/relationship/sex appeal. I don't want to discourage anyone from wearing locks, but you should be aware that these attitudes exist.

Survival Strategies

You will get the brunt of the pestering during your transition period, when you are starting your locks. Here are some suggestions to help you through that period and other situations.

≈≈ You will encounter many people who will find your hair to be exotic, beautiful, and sexy. Sometimes strangers will want to touch your hair. It can get tiresome being a hair ambassador, but look at it this way—they could be throwing eggs. I don't recommend letting strangers touch you or your hair. You can usually tell the difference between someone who is crowding your space and a woman who is genuinely interested in getting a natural style. Try to keep a good humor about it, but be careful.

≈≈ There are plenty of folks wearing locks who are gainfully employed and they are not all entertainers or artists. How about teachers, midwives, attorneys, and psychiatrists, to name a few. But you may want to streamline your appearance at first. For example, long locks can be pinned up into a chignon. Or you may want to postpone starting locks until you are secure in your position. There will be jobs or career opportunities where locks are not going to be accepted, but a short natural will pass muster. Use good judgment and common sense.

There have been reports of tourists wearing locks being scrutinized and even denied entry into some Caribbean countries. During my honeymoon in Freeport, Bahamas, my husband and I saw a sign posted in a movie theater that read NO SHORTS, NO BARE FEET, NO BRAIDS. This is an outrage, but nevertheless. When in doubt, try to check it out with your travel agent or Immigration. It might not be a bad idea to carry a scarf.

Have your locks professionally styled and maintained, if you possibly can. Even if it means traveling to the nearest major city to find the best stylists, it is well worth the trip. Make it a monthly treat—have lunch, see a play or something. A good freelance stylist or locktician is also worth seeing regularly. I can't stress this enough. You'll look and feel so much better after you've been exposed to attractive, successful people with Afrocentric hair. Visiting a good locktician serves the same purpose as patronizing a "straight" salon: It's a feminine ritual that reaffirms your sense of beauty. But don't forget, you'll still need to keep up with your own hair between visits.

Reinforce yourself with the image of attractive locks. Buy and read Afrocentric hair-care magazines. Collect photographs of people with great-looking locks.

Collect beautiful hair accessories. Hair sticks, clips, or ties. Beautiful scarves to tie up your hair. Chic hats to protect your locks from cold winters and shade them from the sun.

Treat yourself to your favorite hair oils. Collect unique jars or bottles to store them in.

Establish a grooming ritual to maintain your locks between visits to your stylist.

≋≋ Corporate Life

If you work in corporate America and are worried about appearances, check out Goddess Braids. They can be as simple as one single braid circling the crown of your head. Cornrows or flat twists done with synthetic extensions can also be done in a conservative, office-smart manner. You and your stylist can think of other suggestions. Keep an open mind.

KEEP YOUR HEAD UP!

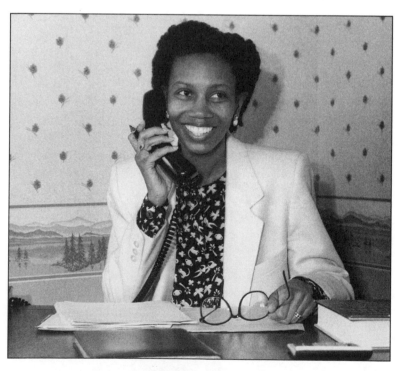

Chauser Perkins Trass, the girl can't help but be professional. She works for the Feds, but it doesn't stop her from working those two-strand twists. And you thought it couldn't be done . . .

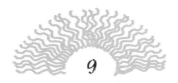

9

Nappy Edges

Braid care is surrounded by a lot of folklore. One popular story is that braids allow you to do nothing with your hair for months at a time. You embark on a sort of hair sabbatical as a reward for the six hours you spent in the chair. After three months of carefree living, you undo the plaits—notice the effortless wording here, "undo"— and your hair trails down your back like the African goddess that you naturally are. Time for a reality check.

All Braided Styles Have a Limited Life Span

When you've spent twelve hours and a few hundred dollars on braids, it's only natural to want them to last a long, long time. But when the party's over, you've got to come home. Learn to recognize when that time comes.

The Honeymoon Phase

Your style is kickin' and heads are turning.

The Companion Phase

You've settled into your braids and worn a few different looks. You've been through a few shampoos, a few oil treatments. You can see a little bit of new growth. You may touch up a few loose plaits every once in a while, but your hair still looks good. The braids still look great after a swim.

The Twilight Phase

You begin to notice that you're doing more maintenance just to get back to the Companion Phase. The relief of a shampoo doesn't last as long as it used to. You're buying a lot of braid spray and paying special attention to brands that claim to soothe itching.

The Terminal Phase

Individual braids are suspended from strands of unbraided hair that is all but locked; the cornrows are floating on an inch or two of new growth. You're tired of scratching. People routinely ask how long you've been wearing braids.

Braid Care with Extensions

Most braids with extensions last anywhere from two to three months before the style is past its prime. The smaller the braid, the longer it will last. Individuals last longer than cornrows. Most extension styles can be cleaned with gentle shampooing and a thorough rinse, so if you feel the need to vigorously massage your hair to get it clean, it's probably time to remove your braids.

Remember, if your scalp is extremely flaky, with signs of pus and serious dandruff soon after you get your braids, then you may have to remove them and/or see a dermatologist.

Shampooing Braids with Extensions

Extensions allow you to shampoo without washing away the structure of your plaits. Even so, take care to disturb them as little as possible. It's not a good idea to shampoo styles done with lin extensions, as lin is a wool fiber that has a tendency to draw up after being wet.

Your braider will suggest her own method for keeping your hair clean. Here are some others. They work best if you wash your hair using a detachable showerhead.

≋≋ Cornrows

If your scalp is a bit flaky, take a soft toothbrush and *gently* work up the dander between the rows so it will rinse out more easily. Dilute your shampoo with a little water and put it into a plastic squeeze bottle with a tip that can get between the rows. Gently sluice your cornrows with the shampoo. Using the pads of your fingers, gently massage the soap into your scalp. Rinse your hair by flooding your cornrows with a gentle flow of water from the showerhead. It is important not to blast your braids with a strong flow of water because you don't want to mat them. You only want to rinse away as much of the dirt as possible. A five-minute rinse is a good idea. Blot excess water from your cornrows with a towel and apply a leave-in conditioner.

You can also protect your braids by shampooing, then covering your hair with a stocking cap while rinsing. You can make a stocking cap by cutting off the leg of a stocking (panty hose aren't suitable for this) at midthigh. Knot the end opposite from the band to form a cap.

As your cornrows age, you may notice a fuzzy halo around them that seems to stop where your own hair ends. This could indicate a couple of things—either you've been lazy about tying your hair up at night or your braids are reaching the Twilight Phase. You may be tempted to do things like shave or cut the fuzzy hair peeking out of the rows. Don't do it! You'll only be cutting your own hair. After shampooing and conditioning, rub a little oil between your palms and smooth it over your hair. Take a satin or silk scarf—for smoothing, a satiny weave is better—tie it down tightly over your hair, and let it air-dry. The scarf helps to tame down the nappy fuzz. When the scarf trick stops working, it's time to make another braid appointment.

≋≋ Individual Braids with Extensions

Use plastic clips to separate your braids into sections for shampooing. Dilute shampoo with a little water and put it into a plastic squeeze bottle with a tip that can get between the parts in your scalp. Gently sluice your scalp with the shampoo. Using low water pressure, saturate your scalp and braids. Gently massage the shampoo through your scalp. Squeeze the suds down the length of the braids in one direction, as if you were laundering a finely knit sweater. You want to clean the braids without disturbing the braid pattern. Finally, rinse the section, using gentle water flow from the showerhead. Shampoo the other sections in the same manner.

Blot your hair dry with a towel and use a leave-in conditioner. Air-dry.

You can also protect your braids by shampooing, then covering your hair with a stocking cap while rinsing.

Shampooing Braids Without Extensions

When your hair is twisted or braided without extensions, it tends to loosen up while it is wet and contract, or tighten, when it dries. Extensions seem to minimize this tendency, and that's why

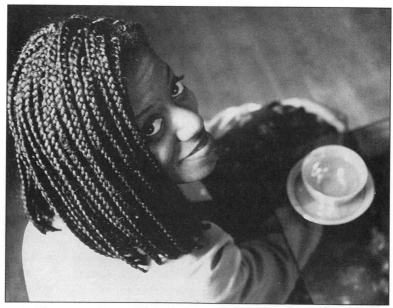

No posing, no primping. Thea just looked up into the camera and it came out like this—gorgeous. On top of that, she can take her braids out in forty minutes.

you can wet most extended styles. It is much more difficult to remove water-tightened braids without extensions; the water encourages them to mat. Therefore, styles braided without extensions are designed to be worn for two or three weeks at a time, then removed.

Cornrows, flat twists, and small individual braids will not survive a shampoo. Plan on taking them down and giving your scalp a good washing.

You can try to shampoo individual twists using the technique described to clean individual braids. But they will draw up or contract after shampooing, depending upon your hair texture. The contraction *may* cause some tangling when it's time to remove your twists, so take extra care when you unfurl them.

Maintaining a Profile of Style

Thea Cook has been wearing braids for more than ten years. Individuals work with her corporate look—suits, skirt sets, or dresses—and they make sense for her exercise workouts. She is a surgery scheduler at a hospital in Los Angeles who is completing a nursing degree. She is also a wife and mother, so her plate is full and there's no time to waste worrying about her hair care. Braids streamline her beauty ritual.

Thea wears individuals for three months at a time. Then she'll give her hair a rest and wear it out for a few weeks before plaiting it up again. She prefers the natural texture of her own shoulder-length hair. She has her braids professionally done by her niece, who happens to be a professional braider/stylist.

While her hair is up, she shampoos every two weeks, since shampooing too frequently dries out her scalp and braids. She uses conditioning oils and braid sprays to keep her scalp and plaits supple. She'll rinse her braids in the shower to keep them fresh between shampoos.

Since her braids are a medium/small size, it only takes forty minutes to remove them. (Girl! You'd better stop telling those lies . . .)

"I'm very focused," she said. "When I know I have to get it

done, I just *do* it." (Actually, this is true—remember, the larger the plait, the less time it takes to undo.)

Thea said she has also worn smaller individuals that were more versatile style wise, but they took about ten hours to remove. (Now, I know *that's* right!)

The Great Shampoo Debate

I used to become irritated when I would wear braids and people would ask, "Can you wash your hair with those in?" Since I wore braids with extensions and washed my hair whenever it seemed dirty, I took this as an affront, as if they were implying that an African-oriented style was less clean than a Eurocentric style. Then I started hearing braiders suggest that braids looked better longer if you shampooed as little as possible. For me, this was easier said than done.

I had my hair done in individual twists without extensions. The stylist said the twists would last for two months before they needed to be redone. This sounded like a long time to me, especially since I knew that braids without extensions were good for two or three weeks at the most. I asked about shampooing and the stylist suggested that I "deep-clean" my scalp in order to preserve the twists as long as possible. She explained that deep cleaning involved moistening a cotton pad with witch hazel or Sea Breeze antiseptic and cleaning the scalp exposed by the parts between my twists. I should also take an antiseptic-moistened pad and run it through the length of my hair, twist by twist. Then I could oil it or use a leave-in conditioner afterward. Couldn't I just shampoo? I asked. Not unless I wanted the twists to draw up, she said. In that case, I'd give the deep cleaning a try.

About two weeks later, my scalp began to itch. It was probably dry, I told myself, and so I oiled it with some scalp conditioner I had gotten from my stylist. It tingled and felt better. Then in another two days, the itching started again. I got out a big bottle of witch hazel and commenced dry washing my scalp with cotton pads, followed by another lube session. The next day, the same areas began to itch again. I replaced the witch hazel with Sea Breeze and did a deep, deep cleaning. By the third week I became self-conscious about standing in front of anyone in the grocery store line because I suspected they might be staring at my scalp. I tried not to scratch in public.

Did I mention that my hair itched? I sat in the bathroom, using hand mirrors to peer at the tender spots on my scalp. Could I have contracted ringworm? Scabies? Eczema? Psoriasis? Could

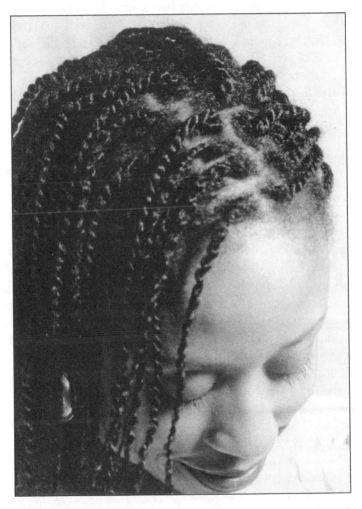

My two-strand twists after I broke down, shampooed, and retwisted them. I'm bowing my head in thanks because the itching finally stopped . . .

one get psoriasis from wearing braids? My husband became concerned.

"Baby, you're scratching like you need a flea collar. Maybe you need to take those twists out."

Our son, Daddy's Little Sidekick, backed him up.

"Fee cower!"

I didn't want to hear that. My *twists* were fine; my *scalp* was the problem. I went to the beauty supply and checked out the braid sprays that I'd claimed were bogus and unnecessary. I bought two bottles and gave my head a good dousing, with extra squirts for the bad spots.

By the next day, it was back like an old refrain.

> Oh, the itch came back,
> The very next day.
> The itch came back.
> I thought it was a goner but—
> The itch came back,
> It just wouldn't stay a-wa-a-y . . .

That was it. I liked my twists, but the itching was unbearable. I felt ridiculous. Twists or no twists, I was going to wash my hair with soap and water and that was all there was to it. Relief at last! My twists did draw up a bit, but it was no big deal. I retwisted the loose areas and kept on stepping.

I don't want to knock the deep clean just because I couldn't hold out. Each scalp is different. Some ladies are able to get by without putting water on their scalp for weeks at a time. A lady told me that she wore braids with extensions for almost three months without washing her hair. When it itched, she used braid spray and it went away. I was suspicious: no smell, no—dare I say it—*itching?* Sure, it itched, she said, but she just kept spraying and it went away.

Deep cleaning and braid sprays are only going to work for so long. There are even sprays marketed as "braid shampoos," which are formulated with ingredients like sulfur. (If your hair has been chemically straightened, most experts recommend avoiding preparations containing sulfur.) Don't let the prospect of having to remove your braids prevent you from using common sense. Some scalps function well with a monthly shampoo. Others can go longer. Still others can't take it after a week. If your hair feels nasty, wash it.

Oils

Itching is usually caused by a dry scalp, so try to moisturize or lubricate the problem away before you reach for the dandruff remedies. Hot-oil treatments are very effective. You can buy oils at health-food stores or beauty suppliers. Here's one formula I use:

¼ cup olive oil (good lubricant)
1 tsp. rosemary oil (promotes smoothing of the cuticle)
½ tsp. sage oil (alleviates itching)

Mix oils. Dampen your braids or cornrows. Heat oil to a comfortable temperature before applying to hair ends and scalp. Cover braids with a plastic cap. Warm your hair with an electric heating cap for twenty minutes or cover the plastic cap with a thick towel for forty minutes. Shampoo and apply a leave-in conditioner.

If you suspect you have dandruff, try a mild dandruff shampoo. Shampoo suggestions are included in the section on dandruff in Chapter 2, "Four Degrees of Preparation."

You can also lubricate your braids and twists with natural oils. You can try commercial preparations or mixing small amounts of your own recipes. For instance, try olive or almond oil as a base, and add a couple of drops of oils like rosemary, aloe vera, jojoba, bergamot, or nettle (herb) extract. Aloe vera and sage oils are good for itchy scalps. You can find oils and herbs at a good health store. Pour a little in your hands, rub them together, and rub it into your braids or use sparingly on your scalp. The key phrase here is *use oils in a sparing manner.* You don't want to overload your scalp with large doses of oil, nor do you want your braids to become saturated. It's a good idea to purchase small amounts of oils and keep them in a cool place, away from direct sunlight.

Commercial oil lotions like Luster's Pink Oil Lotion are effective, but you'll have to take care to work them into your hair gently so they don't leave a visible residue or film.

Braid Sprays

Most braid sprays are designed to moisturize the scalp, which minimizes itching and puts a sheen on your braids. Glycerine, a humectant that absorbs moisture from the air, is a main ingredient. It's also the same ingredient used in curly perm moisturizers and curl activators. Braid sprays and liquids that promise shine can include silicone-based ingredients. They physically smooth the cuticle and deposit a sheen of silicone oil. If you rely solely upon braid spray to lubricate your hair, you'd best stock up. The effects of braid sprays and/or sheen products are short-lived. Glycerine buildup can be a bit sticky; if you plan on using a lot of these products, it's best to give your hair a daily rinse. I prefer using a braid spray only if my hair is parched and I don't have time for a hot-oil treatment.

Nighttime Care

Your braids will look fresher longer if you cover them with a scarf before you nap or go to bed at night. Satin or tightly woven silk is the best choice to smooth down braids and cornrows. Cotton scarves tend to absorb protective oils and encourage the fuzzies. For extra insurance, pick up a satin pillow cover—you can get one for a few dollars—in case you sleep restlessly and your scarf ends up at the foot of your bed in the morning.

Place your braids in the direction you want them to lie before you tie your scarf and you won't have wayward plaits in the morning. If you do wake up with a wild braid or two, a light spritz of water or braid spray will tame them.

The Right Tools

You'll want to change your look from time to time, and using hair accessories is an obvious way to do that, but it's important that you make the *right* choice. The idea here is to use aids and accessories that don't encourage the breakage cycle.

≋ Hair Accessories

Braids, twists, and locks can work wonders, but if you continue to use metal hair implements like bobby pins, barrettes, clips, and the like, your hair will soon tell on you. The edges of the metal clips rub against your hair shaft like little knives, which weakens and breaks the shafts off. Jettison those banana clips or any other

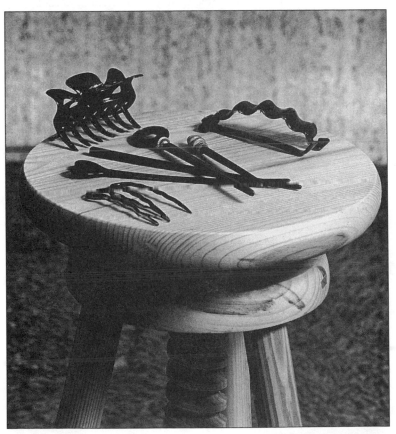

These hair sticks, clasps, and faux tortoiseshell hair pins will be gentle adornment to your braids, locks, and twists. Remember, avoid materials that will damage your hair.

clip or barrette with teeth; they wreak havoc on braids and twists. I know it is tempting to pull those long braids back into a clip. Just be careful about how the clip is made.

≋≋ Better Choice

Hair sticks, faux tortoiseshell hair pins, and clips with smooth edges and no metal parts. You can find them at barrette displays in beauty supply stores, better department stores, and those little accessory boutiques in shopping malls. Barrettes fashioned with a plastic cover and a small stick that pokes through are a good choice, as are fabric ponytail holders made of satin or silky material.

Touch-Ups

First, the good news—individual two-strand twists done without extensions are a snap to touch up. If you've done your own, there's no problem. If a braider has done yours for you, just follow her original partings—"the grid"—and redo each twist, one by one. Be sure and twist in the same direction.

If the ends of your braids unravel, you can carefully rebraid, taking care to keep your braid pattern tight. Most braiders will seal synthetic extensions by burning the ends with a lighter and rolling the tips between the fingers. Some braiders knot the ends before burning. (If you try this, please put the lighter on the lowest flame setting and watch your fingers.) Others simply braid the ends tightly. Other methods include dipping the ends in hot water or bumping them with a curling iron for styling effects.

Now the bad news. Unless you know how to braid, you can forget about repairing individual extensions and cornrows. Your attempt is bound to look crooked and amateurish next to a professional's work. Consult your braider about a touch-up or make an appointment for a new set of braids.

Everything Must Change

Braids are so convenient that many ladies have embraced them for life. That's well and good, but after a year of wearing the same braid extension style, parted in the exact same areas, you may notice some changes. Your side part is becoming wider and wider and your hairline is creeping back farther and farther.

You must change your braid style regularly or traction alopecia will take your hair out. Find an alternative braid style or change the partings. You can even wear your hair in thick Goddess Braids if you can't bear to be without some type of braids, but give your hairline a break.

Sporting Braids

Braids and twists are extremely practical for athletically minded women or health club workouts. They are a great choice for sweat-producing activities, like track or basketball, that leave hair standing on top of your head.

After working out, if your scalp is really sweaty, you have a few options: If you're pressed for time, swab your parts with Sea Breeze and spritz with braid spray. If you have a little more time, do a quick, light shampoo and use a leave-in conditioner.

Braided styles using extensions are almost perfect for swimming. You can even get away with swimming in braids or cornrows done without extensions if you keep the sections large, to minimize the possibility of matting. Large sections also make the hair easier to take down, so it can be thoroughly shampooed.

After swimming, be sure to rinse your hair thoroughly in fresh water, then shampoo and chase it with a leave-in conditioner. The last thing you need is chlorine or saltwater deposits lodged in your plaits.

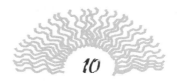

10

The Promised Land

There's no use in glossing over reality here. Think about the mornings that you rose out of bed and took off for the office. The weekends that you slept in late, shook out your hair, and rushed out to brunch. The rainy days when you watched your friends with perms run for cover. You're going to pay for them when it's time to take your braids down.

Taking It Down—
A Long Day's Work

As a general rule, it will take at least as long to take your braids down as it took to put them in. Styles using extensions take longer to remove and individuals with extensions are especially labor intensive. That's just the price you pay for the versatility of individuals. Plan on an entire weekend for most braid jobs. If it took twelve hours to put individuals in, plan on two or three days to remove them without assistance. This doesn't count shampooing, conditioning, or trims.

Braids *without* extensions take less time, but individuals are going to take more. Cornrows without extensions are not difficult to remove. Two-strand twists—even individuals, in my experience—are no problem. However, and this is a big "however," taking down hair that has been braided without extensions and shampooed is a different story. If your hair has drawn up after the shampoo and the braids are small, chances are that you're going to have a major job on your hands trying to take them out. You may need the help of a friend or a professional if the ends of the plaits have become slightly meshed. It's not an impossible job, but you have been warned.

The first time I took my cornbraids down, I thought about putting a contract out on the braider. All kidding aside, I was not up to the task. Oh, I thought I was, but I really had no idea what I was in for.

I had one layer of cornbraids with extensions that trailed past my shoulders. It took about six hours to put them in. It took *two days* to take them out. I wasn't sure where my own hair started and the extension hair began, so I was afraid of trimming too much of it away. My fingers cramped up pulling masses of shedded hair and caked dandruff, dandruff that didn't show while the cornrows were in, but sho' nuff made an appearance when the extensions came out. It seemed like it took the better part of an hour to get two rows out.

Then there was the matter of my nappy new hair. Straight out of the plaits, it was as if my crop had been paroled after a long sentence and didn't know what to do first. It was dirty and I was too tired to even consider a shampoo. I wrestled it down with a brush and mumbled something about getting it into a bun for the time being. My hair just laughed and said, "I don't think so."

So I hopped into the shower. When I had shampooed my braids, my own hair would try to coil but the extensions prevented total contraction. These were the days before I knew how to minimize tangling during a shampoo. As soon as the water hit my newly freed hair, that was all she wrote. It drew up like a parched jheri curl. I grabbed some balsam conditioner (I didn't know any better) and tried to soften it up. Spent another three hours trying to comb it out and blow it dry. My arms ached and my scalp was sore. I tried to console myself that all the hair at my feet had come from shedding and not from pulling it through snarls and knots.

After a year of braiding, my hair had grown the fabled six inches that all the books and doctors say it should have, but that first session was a test in every sense of the word. I learned the hard way. You don't have to.

≋ Removing Extensions–The Quick Method

Everyone's looking for that hook up, that quick way out. Forget about it. We've heard about the braid sprays that are designed to remove extensions and weaves. If you like them, try them. I don't have a problem with it. I also don't see any little people coming out of the bottle and undoing the braids. By the time you get to your ninth straight hour of unplaiting, you may indeed see little people crawling out of your braid spray, and if they help you get through it—more power to you. For my money, the smarter move is to get the spray—and two or three of your friends. Take all of them home and let them help you remove your braids.

≋ How to Remove Long Extensions–The Real Method

Spread some newspaper around your work area and grab a wastebasket with plastic liner bags, which you can use to dispose of the hair. Please, throw it away. Some ladies are tempted to try and save human hair if they've spent a little change on it. Believe me, you'll be happy to see it go. You'll also need a rattailed comb, a wide-toothed comb, hair scissors, braid spray (if you like it), and plastic clips to divide your hair into sections and keep the unbraided hair in check.

≋ Removing Long Individual Extensions

Divide your braids into manageable sections. Remember how long your hair was before you put it up? Take a fist full of braids, measure about three inches below that, and cut the extension. It should start to unravel immediately, allowing you to unbraid it. You can use the tail end of the rat comb to help it along.

When you get to the base knot, where the extension has been added, the false hair should slide out with no problem. Even though you may have shampooed while your hair was up, still a certain amount of oil, dirt, dandruff, or shed scalp cells will be trapped at the base of your extensions. This is natural, so don't become alarmed. If there is a lot of dirt lodged in the base knot, work the tail of the comb through the knot to loosen it. If the hair is terribly matted, try a little braid spray to loosen it. Be patient and work through it. Try to remember that tearing your hair out at the root will only earn you a bald spot, so it is worth your time to see it through. If the knot seems impossible, this is where your friends come in. You can also consult your braider.

As you remove the braids from each fist-sized section, comb through it with the wide-toothed comb. You'll notice a lot of hair coming out with the dirt. This is hair that has been shed while your hair was up but stayed there because it was held in by the plaits. The longer your hair was up, the more shed hair you'll have, so again, don't be alarmed. In fact, even women with fine hair should notice that their hair seems thick and healthy in the root area, even after clearing away masses of shedded hair. Shiny, bald spots or radical thinning call for a dermatologist's help.

≋ Removing Cornbraids and Cornrows

If your cornbraids are in layers, measure three inches below where you think your hair ends and trim the braids, working up through the cornrowed area. You can remove them in the same manner as with the individuals. If you have cornrows, I don't recommend trimming because your own hair is woven into each row in such a way that makes it difficult to know whose hair you're cutting. Cornrows are a bit easier to remove, anyway.

≋ Removing Twists Without Extensions

For me, these are the easiest sell. Less time to put in, easier to take down. Give the base of the twist a slight turn in the opposite direction that it was twisted in. Hook a finger between the two strands at the base and unfurl the twist. Separate and comb out in the same manner as you would if removing three-strand braids.

≋ Removing Twists with Extensions

Since the extension is anchored with a base knot, you'll have to work from the end. Trim the extension down in the same manner used for braid extensions. Unfurl the twist. Separate and comb out shed hair and section off for shampooing.

≋ Removing Silky Locks

This suggestion is for locks that are created by wrapping synthetic hair around a braided extension base. Examine the base (root) of the lock. If thread has been used to anchor it, you should enlist a friend to help remove the thread because chances are great that you will cut your own hair by mistake if you try removing the thread unassisted. You can try removing them by cutting the tip off the end of the lock. Unravel the extension wrap from the braided base and remove. Then remove the braided extension in the manner previously described.

≋ Shampooing After Braid Removal

After your braids are out, keep your hair sectioned off. Then give it a thorough comb-out, section by section, to remove as much shedded hair and dirt as you can. Then section your hair for your shampoo. I use a mild cleansing shampoo and follow with a hot-oil treatment. (Suggestions for shampooing are in Chapter 2, "Four Degrees of Preparation.")

Growth Cycles

This is usually where most of us want to be—enjoying the longer and healthier hair that braiding can promote. The braids and twists protect your hair from damage and stress. The hair ends— the oldest and most fragile part—are protected from breakage. So you're more likely to actually see the growth that would otherwise be unnoticeable after a month of gradual breakage.

Human hair grows an average of half an inch a month. There are three stages to the cycle. In the *catogen* phase, the new hair prepares to emerge from its follicle. The growth phase is called the *anogen,* or active, period, which can be as long as three years. The resting stage is the *telogen* period, after which the hair is shed and a new growth cycle begins. On average, there are about 80,000 to 150,000 hairs per scalp.

One last caveat. Beware of braiders who want to charge you a price based upon the amount of extensions they use. Unless you're purchasing some wildly expensive hair blessed by Nefertiti herself, the hair should be included in the deal. I witnessed the result of too much of a good thing when a friend of mine returned from a stay in Kenya. My friend, whose name has been deleted to protect our friendship, returned to the United States with what I had been told was a fabulous head of braids, done by a braider in Mombasa. I couldn't wait to see her.

Family and friends were gathered for a welcome-home dinner. And there was our homegirl, braids adorned with—a very chic scarf from Kenya.

"Hey, girl! Lemme see that hair!" I said, and made an unsuccessful grab for the scarf.

"All in good time," she said, pulling me and two other friends into a bedroom. What was up?

The scarf came off. She had already begun removing some braids, but the rest, at least at first glance, appeared to be okay. Why did she want to take them out so quickly?

"Girl, I've been trying to get these out for the last couple of days." Couple of days? I took a closer look. Wow. Girlfriend had never been hurting for hair to begin with, but now it was . . . rather abundant.

Somebody grabbed a wastebasket and the four of us got busy. After we'd emptied the first of three small baskets in less than thirty minutes, it was obvious that homegirl was holding out on us. Did I mention that girlfriend's braids seemed plentiful? I myself wondered why she hadn't been detained at Customs, on suspicion of attempting to smuggle extension hair into the United States.

After we threatened to stop helping her unless she 'fessed up, the real story came out. It turns out that the braiders in Mombasa based their fee on the amount of hair they used on the client's head. In girlfriend's case, three braiders working together used eight packages of extensions. Eight. And this wasn't any French Refined, either. It was, oh, Barbie Plus. Talk about a profit incentive. "Here at SmorgaBraids, we give you as much hair as your neck can support."

The extensions were heavy as all get-out, itchy and uncomfortable, but she gave it her best. She shampooed. She conditioned. Then she shampooed and conditioned again. But it was all to no avail. It was just too much.

Actually, it was a lot of fun helping her take them out and it took maybe an hour and a half. If you have a lot to take down, it definitely helps to have friends.

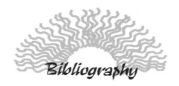

Bibliography

Africa Adorned, by Angela Fisher. New York: Harry N. Abrams, Inc., 1984.

African Hairstyles, by Esi Sagay. Portsmouth, N.H.: Heinemann Educational Books, Inc., 1985.

A Consumer's Dictionary of Cosmetic Ingredients, by Ruth Winter. New York: Crown Publishers, 1989.

Curly Hair, by Willie Lee Morrow. San Diego, Calif.: Black Publishers of San Diego, a division of Willie Morrow Unlimited, Inc., 1973.

Daring Do's, by Mary Trasko. Paris: Flammarion, 1994.

Everything You Need to Know About Hairlocking, by Nekhena Evans. Brooklyn, N.Y.: New Bein' Press, 1993.

Milady's Black Cosmetology, by Thomas Hayden and James Williams. Albany, N.Y.: Milady Publishing Company, 1990.

Photograph and Illustration Credits

Pages 14–15: Photographs courtesy of Raziya Al-Nafis

Pages 16–17, 19: Photographs by Aurelio Jose Barrera

Pages 26, 74–78, 85, 90–91: Illustrations by P. J.

Pages 28–29: Illustrations by Sergei Loobkoff

Page 55: Photograph of Lonnice Brittenum Bonner by Laura J. Brooks. Hair by Queen Raziya.

Pages 61 & 107: Photographs courtesy of Lonnice Brittenum Bonner

Page 62: Photograph courtesy of Lonnice Brittenum Bonner. Braids by Maxine Jones.

Page 93: Photograph by Aurelio Jose Barrera. Hair by Connie.

Page 94: Photograph by Aurelio Jose Barrera. Hair by Raziya Al-Nafis.

Page 95: Photograph courtesy of Raziya Al-Nafis. Hair by Raziya Al-Nafis.

Page 100: Photograph by Lauren Lee Salgaller. Hair by Chauser Perkins Trass.

Page 104: Photograph by Aurelio Jose Barrera. Hair by Ayana Williams.

Page 107: Photograph by Laura J. Brooks

Page 111: Accessories courtesy of Lonnice Brittenum Bonner. Photo by Laura J. Brooks.

Lonnice Brittenum Bonner's two-strand twists and Capril Bonner-Thomas's locks were styled by:

Queen Raziya
Inglewood, Calif.
310-671-6765

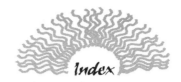

Index